GROUP WORK WITH OLDER ADULTS

85 Therapeutic Exercises for Reminiscence, Validation, and Remotivation

ANN L. LINK

Professional Resource Press
Sarasota, Florida

Published by Professional Resource Press
(An Imprint of Professional Resource Exchange, Inc.)
Post Office Box 3197
Sarasota, FL 34230-3197
www.prpress.com

Printed in the United States of America

To order:
Professional Resource Press
PO Box 3197
Sarasota, FL 34230-3197
Tel: (800) 443-3364
Fax: (866) 804-4843
Online: www.prpress.com
E-mail: cs.prpress@gmail.com

Library of Congress Cataloging-in-Publication Data

Link, Ann L., date.
Group work with older adults : 85 therapeutic exercises for reminiscence, validation, and remotivation / Ann L. Link.
pages cm
Includes bibliographical references.
ISBN-13: 978-1-56887-149-3
ISBN-10: 1-56887-149-X
1. Group psychotherapy for older people. 2. Occupational therapy for older people. 3. Social work with older people. I. Title.
RC451.4.A5L556 2014
618.97'89152--dc23

2013031728

Let's Talk

I roam a landscape of the past,
I wander hallways looking for a friend.
I turn a corner, try a door,
I whisper secrets as I pace the floor.
I long for a familiar smile,
I hide my loneliness behind a yawn.
Come talk with me a little while,
Let's share some tales
Before the day is gone.

Ann Link

DEDICATION

With love and appreciation to my

parents, family, supportive friends,

and elder group members

TABLE OF CONTENTS

INTRODUCTION

PURPOSE OF THE BOOK

Group Work With Older Adults offers 85 exercises to broaden group topics relevant to aging. Some of these exercises have been updated from those that appeared in Dr. Link's earlier publication, *Group Work With Elders*, published in 1997. Many are brand new. This book is designed to aid therapists and trained group facilitators who conduct discussion groups for geriatric clients. Exercises in the book combine important geriatric therapy techniques of Reminiscence, Validation, and Remotivation to energize group discussion and foster renewal of hope.

Group participation is a therapeutic tool which is widely supported by experts in the field of geriatrics (Haight & Gibson, 2005). Structured exercises and instructions for group leaders in this book focus on issues pertinent to the aging process such as coping with loss, physical illness, and decline in independence. Illustrated handouts increase opportunities for participation among group members who have varying levels of cognitive and physical functioning.

BENEFITS OF GROUP

Curative elements of group work described by Yalom and Molyn (1995) apply to elder populations. The benefits of catharsis, universality, guidance, instillation of hope, group cohesiveness, and interpersonal learning are especially valuable to older group members. Illness, loss of loved ones, and declines in independence increase the likelihood of depression, isolation, and diminished self-worth. Group therapy provides beneficial social interaction, support in coping with frustration, and validation of feelings (Husaini et al., 2004). In many cases, group participation helps to reduce isolation and lack of relatedness. The exercises are designed to increase feelings of belonging and community. Group members who have a reduced sense of identity and experience confusion may strengthen their reality focus and coping skills through group participation.

SPECIFIC THERAPEUTIC USES OF THE EXERCISES

VENTILATION AND VALIDATION OF FEELINGS

Group participation helps to validate and affirm feelings and experiences of older adults (Toseland, 1990). Interacting with peers who express similar concerns and emotional reactions encourages group members in their efforts to cope with adverse life experiences. Feeling heard, understood, and accepted are major building blocks to self-esteem in the elderly. Relating to the emotional tone of communication is often more important than focusing on content (Feil & Klerk-Rubin, 2002).

Many exercises encourage artistic expression which enhances communication and is therapeutic for emotional pain and suffering. Depending on their limitations, some members may be able to communicate more fully by using colors or drawing to express their feelings which can be a healing experience. There is not a solution or cure for many challenges of old age, but healing can still continue on an emotional and spiritual level (Malchiodi, 2002).

REMINISCENCE

Many exercises in this book are designed to trigger reminiscence, which is a valuable tool in helping the elderly client review life events to gain perspective, derive meaning, and work toward resolution (Haight & Gibson, 2005). Erickson (1998) describes the tasks of later life as developing integrity and wisdom versus despair. Research has shown that group reminiscence therapy reduces depression and increases cognitive function (Wang, 2007). Relating to others in a meaningful way is important stimulation for the brain. Members share past accomplishments, explore disappointments, and arrive at new viewpoints.

REMOTIVATION AND INSTILLATION OF HOPE

The older adult in a residual setting often has difficulty investing interest in his or her present environment, which leads to feelings of isolation and hopelessness. During supportive group interaction, members become better acquainted with each other and increase their awareness of possible interests and activities available in their living situation. Positive group interaction can increase self-esteem, motivation, and a sense of hope (Dyer & Stotts, 2005).

INTERPERSONAL LEARNING

Coping with stress is a never-ending life task. Reviewing past coping skills encourages members in their efforts to deal with frustration and adapt to change (Toseland, 1990). Listening to others in a group describe coping skills and survival techniques promotes interpersonal learning. We now understand that the brain has a property called neuroplasticity, the ability to change its structure and patterns of activity in significant ways not only in childhood, but also in adulthood and throughout life (Davidson & Begley, 2012). Opportunities are presented in the exercises to learn coping behaviors in a supportive atmosphere. Members are encouraged to think of solutions to problems in a new way.

GROUP COHESION AND RELATEDNESS

Loss of loved ones and weakening of social ties often lead to feelings of worthlessness and isolation for the elderly. Making new connections with people is difficult; however, feelings of relatedness and belonging enhance self-esteem and increase motivation for living. Group provides the opportunity to offer altruistic support to others which increases feelings of self-worth (Agronin, 2009). The exercises presented in this book are designed to foster group cohesion and interaction in a nonthreatening, therapeutic format.

SUGGESTIONS AND PRECAUTIONS FOR GROUP LEADERS

INTRODUCTION TO THE GROUP

Many elders may not be open to the idea of a mental health therapy group, feeling that there is a stigma attached to participation. Members often prefer to call the group a "class" or simply a "discussion group." The purpose of the group might be explained as an opportunity to become better acquainted, share ideas, and learn from each other's experiences.

SELECTION OF MEMBERS

Although a structured group process can sustain varying levels of cognitive functioning and is beneficial for many elders, it is not appropriate for everyone. Group participation may be counterproductive for highly disruptive individuals, persons who cannot allow others to have their turn at speaking, or members who wander off while the group is in session.

GROUP SETTING

Seating around a square or round table where members can see each other is recommended. A private or semiprivate atmosphere encourages disclosure. Some group leaders include a snack or beverage at the end of the session to encourage relatedness and a sense of belonging.

GROUP FORMAT

Structured group formats are often effective for geriatric populations because they generate interaction, provide focus, stimulate reminiscence, and promote inclusion. Flexibility should allow for unstructured discussion as well. Some leaders alternate structured groups with unstructured groups. Other leaders allow time at the beginning of each group session to deal with immediate concerns of group members, such as illness, situational events, natural disasters, and so forth. It is important to stay in touch with the needs of group members to ensure that the group experience is relevant and valuable.

CONFIDENTIALITY

Members are encouraged to respect each other's privacy and refrain from revealing information learned within the group to persons outside the group.

GROUP LEADER'S ROLE

Inclusion is very important in working with older adults in groups (Haight & Gibson, 2005). Each member should be welcomed at every session, and members' names should be used profusely throughout the sessions. The leader should be instrumental in preventing any individual from dominating the group. Each member should have an opportunity to contribute to the discussion. Group members should be encouraged, but not pressured, to participate in the exercises. Members need to feel in control of how much or how little they divulge. Each contribution should be acknowledged. Modeling a supportive, accepting attitude while maintaining appropriate boundaries and structure is a key element to successful group leadership and may help members to generalize these attitudes outside of the group.

MEMBERS WITH IMPAIRMENTS

Many groups for the elderly will include members who have some degree of impairment which impedes communication. The goal of the group leader is to enhance individual participation to maximize each member's potential for interaction. It may not be realistic that each member relate to every aspect of an exercise. A more realistic goal is to use techniques in leading the group that maximize each individual's potential for interaction. Some members will benefit from the entire scope of an exercise, while other members may relate only to a portion of the exercise, such as reminiscence connected to the illustration. It is imperative that the leader model an accepting attitude toward individual differences. This is accomplished by focusing on the member's contribution rather than directing attention to some part of the exercise the member has not been able to complete. For example, if a group member declines to complete most of an exercise, but colors some part of the illustration, the leader may encourage interaction by saying something like: "Mary, I notice that you have colored the roof of the well red. I'm wondering if this has some special meaning for you?" Mary, in turn, may respond with reminiscence of a red-roofed well in her past. The feeling tone of colors and drawings can be commented on in a supportive manner, making sure to always check out the validity of impressions with the group member. It is important to emphasize the importance of expression of feelings rather than artistic talent (Malchiodi, 2002). Drawing and color enhance communication, but each exercise can also be used effectively with verbal or written participation.

Some of the exercises have optional suggestions for songs to enhance reminiscence. Research has shown that music is an important stimulant for the brain that significantly improves recall (Larkin, 2001).

Members with memory problems can sometimes relate to a familiar tune or lyric more easily than to illustrations or printed material. Suggestions for accompanying songs are optional and each exercise can also be effectively used without music.

A main function of a therapeutic group is to foster meaningful interaction and a sense of belonging. Exercise sheets are to be used as a guide and stimulus for participation, not as mandatory assignments. Members may fill out as much or as little of an exercise sheet as they desire. Whether or not they read or write, each member is given an exercise sheet as a symbol of inclusion. Words are provided in the exercises for those who like to read and write. In some cases, members respond more fully by writing than by talking. It is important to describe pictures and read sentences aloud to include members who do not see well or cannot read or write. These individuals are included in the discussion as members are encouraged to share their ideas verbally.

Persons who are hard of hearing often appreciate visual and written guidelines included in the exercise sheets. These members may also be seated near the leader to facilitate hearing. It is always important for the leader to speak clearly and distinctly, repeating questions and directions as needed.

CONFUSED OR DELUSIONAL MEMBERS

Severely disturbed individuals who cannot focus and who interrupt others continually are not appropriate for inclusion in a group. Members who are able to focus to some extent and are moderately confused or delusional can benefit from a group if the leader provides appropriate structure and support. Most exercises feature a concrete, familiar topic to help strengthen a reality focus; thus, if a confused group member strays from the topic, bringing up unrelated or delusional ideas, the leader may gently redirect the discussion back to the topic. For example, the leader might respond, "Bob, you have described ideas about spacemen. Today our topic is food. Can you name some foods you like?"

If the delusional response refers to the topic, the leader can show understanding for the feeling tone of the response without directly confirming or disputing the content of the remark. For example, Alice may assert that her mother poisoned the family's bread when she baked. The leader might respond, "Alice, it sounds like you felt distrustful of eating bread your mother baked." The leader may also redirect toward a positive focus by asking questions, such as, "Was there any bread you felt comfortable eating?" or "When did you enjoy eating bread?" Directly disputing a delusional response may cause a member to feel misunderstood and defensive. Acknowledging the emotion behind a delusional statement provides support and encourages communication (Feil & Klerk-Rubin, 2002).

MEMORY PROBLEMS

It is important that the group leader deal with participants' memory problems in a supportive manner to lessen feelings of inadequacy. Several techniques are helpful in maintaining participation when a group member cannot recall something asked for in an exercise. The leader can ask for voluntary responses by asking, "Who would like to share a memory they have about baking bread?" Members who do not respond to this question may be asked related questions that do not require as much memory, such as, "Mary, do you like bread with your meals?" Asking questions in a multiple-choice format helps to trigger memories; for example, the leader may encourage a response by asking, "Bob, what do you like better, home-baked bread or store-bought bread?" (Feil & Klerk-Rubin, 2002).

Another technique that encourages responses is to involve the group. For example, if a member is asked to name a romantic person and responds, "I don't know" or "I don't remember," the leader may ask the group for help by saying, "Who can suggest people Alice may have found romantic?" Suggestions might include Alice's husband, Paul Newman, and so on. The leader then thanks the group for their suggestions and asks Alice if any of the suggestions match her idea of a romantic person. This is a variation on the multiple-choice format that often elicits a response. It is helpful to remember that the most important function of any exercise is to encourage expression and a feeling of belonging.

CONCLUSION

Leading groups for geriatrics is greatly enhanced by use of these exercises. Complex tasks of aging deserve the special emphasis featured in this book. Coming to terms with the meaning of life in its final stages can be lonely and overwhelming. Meeting with others to share feelings, experiences, and ideas for coping reduces isolation and despair. Group facilitators take on the rewarding challenge of inspiring older adults in their psychological struggle to attain integrity and preserve dignity.

REFERENCES

Agronin, M. (2009). Group therapy in older adults. *Current Psychiatry Reports, Feb.; 11*(1): 27-32.

Dyer, J., & Stotts, M. (2005). *Handbook of Remotivation Therapy.* New York: Haworth Clinical Practice Press.

Davidson, R., & Begley, S. (2012). *The Emotional Life of Your Brain.* New York: Hudson Street Press.

Erickson, E. (1998). *The Life Cycle Completed* (ext ver.). New York: W.W. Norton and Company.

Feil, N., & Klerk-Rubin, V. (2002). *The Validation Breakthrough* (3rd ed.) Baltimore, MD: Health Professional Press.

Haight, B., & Gibson, F. (2005) *Working with Older Adults, Group Process and Techniques* (4th ed.). Boston: Jones and Bartlett.

Husaini, B. A., Cummings, S., Kilbourne, B., Roback, H., Sherkat, D., Levine, R., & Cain, V. A. (2004). Group therapy for depressed elderly women. *International Journal of Group Psychotherapy, 54*(3), 295-319.

Larkin, M. (2001). Music tunes up memory in dementia patients. *Lancet, 357*(9249), 47.

Malchiodi, C. (2002). *The Soul's Palette.* Boston, MA: Shambhala Publications.

Toseland, R. (1990). *Group Work with Older Adults.* New York: University Press

Wang, J. J. (2007). Group reminiscence therapy for cognitive and affective function of demented elderly in Taiwan. *International Journal Geriatric Psychiatry, Dec; 22*(12), 1235-1240.

Yalom, I. D., & Molyn, L. (1995). *The Theory and Practice of Group Psychotherapy* (5th ed.). New York: Basic Books.

Exercise 1

SENTIMENTAL JOURNEY

Purpose:

- Share memories about travel to increase feelings of belonging.
- Open up feelings about places and events of the past.

Materials:

A copy of the illustration for each group member; pencils, crayons, or fine-line colored felt pens. ***Optional:*** A recording of the song "Sentimental Journey."

Procedure:

1. Materials are distributed and the sentence fragment is read aloud.
2. Members are asked to describe travel modes and locations in the picture.
3. Members who wish may color the picture or add other details.
4. If available, a recording of the song "Sentimental Journey" is played.

Group Discussion:

Group members are asked to share memories about the song and places they have lived or visited. The group leader encourages members to share about trips made for schooling, vacations, weddings, funerals, or other important life events. Sharing personal history increases group cohesion and reduces isolation.

The group leader asks members to share their pictures and sentences about where they would like to take a sentimental journey and why that trip would have special memories for them. Reminiscence and expression of feelings reduces depression and enhances cognitive functioning.

Sentimental Journey

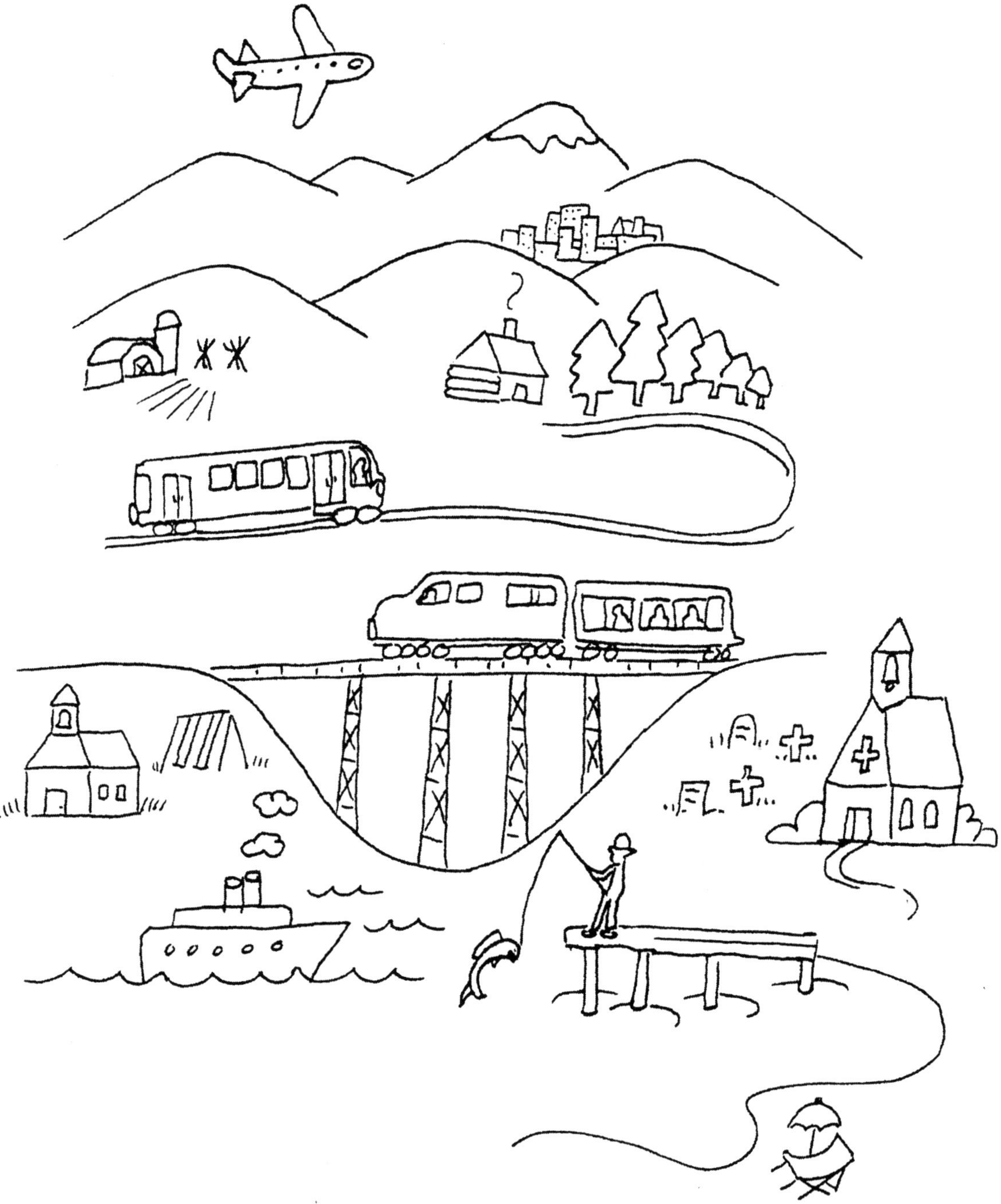

If I took a sentimental journey, I would travel to: ____________

____

____

Exercise 2

COLLECT POSITIVE THOUGHTS

Purpose:

- Discuss the relationship between positive thoughts and moods.
- Share personal information about hobbies to increase feelings of belonging.

Materials:

One photocopy of the illustration for each group member; pencils, crayons, or fine-line colored felt pens.

Procedure:

1. Materials are passed out and the caption is read aloud.
2. Members are asked to think about things they have collected.
3. The sentence fragment is read aloud and members are asked to fill in the blank.
4. Members may draw something they have collected or color the pictures.

Group Discussion:

Members are asked why it is important to make a collection of positive thoughts. Members may recall that negative thoughts contribute to depression and discouragement. The leader points out that practicing positive thoughts has a beneficial effect on one's mood. Negative thoughts increase stress which is not good for a person's health. The leader asks each member to suggest a positive thought for the day.

Members share their sentences and describe something they have collected. Learning more about each other's hobbies and interests helps to reduce isolation and increase feelings of belonging.

Collect Positive Thoughts

Make a collection of positive thoughts.
Store them with care, display them often, and
watch their value increase.

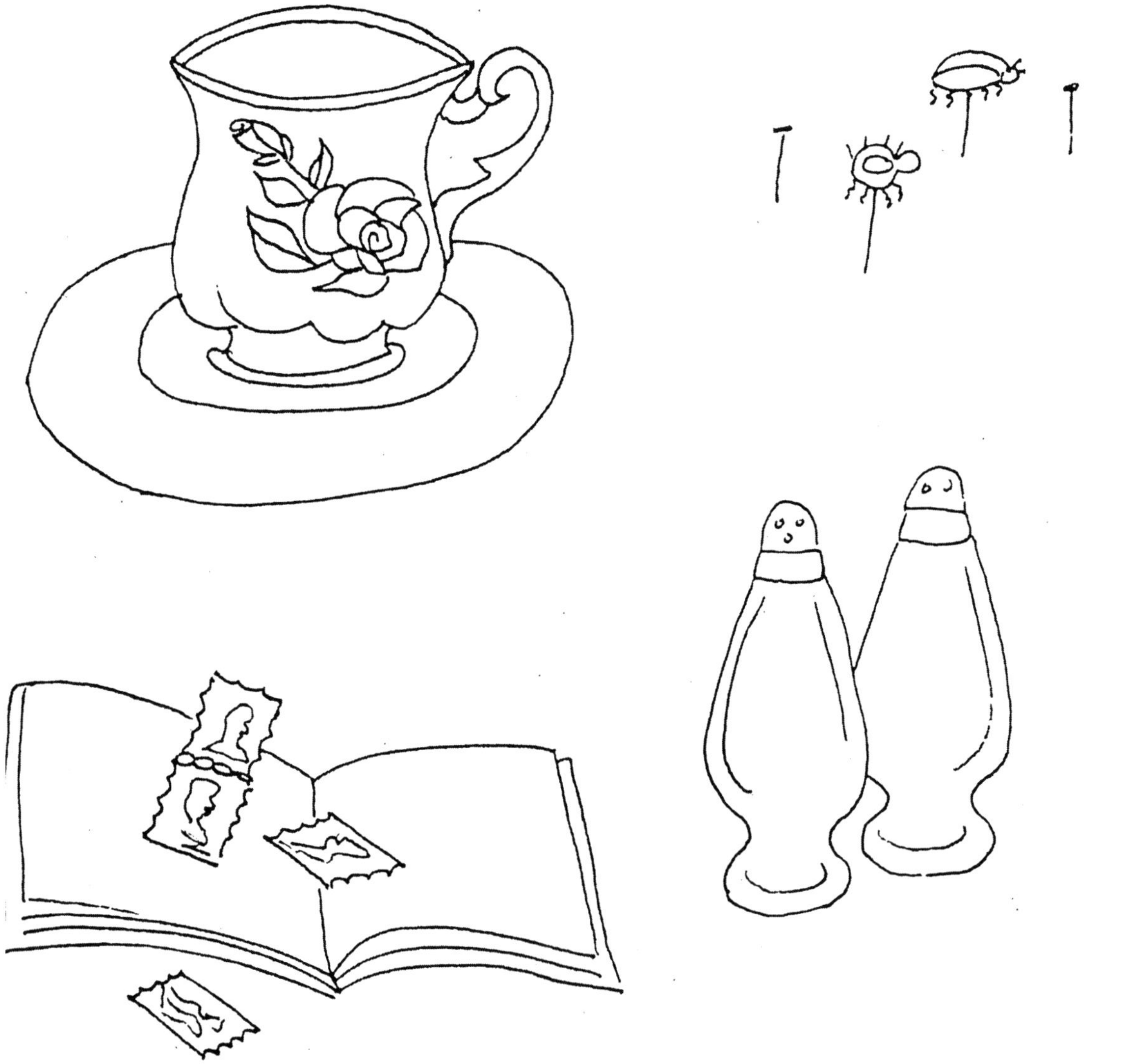

Something I have collected: ______________________

Exercise 3

SOMETHING THAT BUGS ME

Purpose:

- Share frustrations and ideas for coping with annoyances.
- Share personal information to increase group cohesiveness.

Materials:

One photocopy of the illustration for each group member; pencils, crayons, or fine-line colored felt pens.

Procedure:

1. Materials are passed out and the sentence fragment is read aloud.
2. Members are asked to think about things that "bug" them or bother them.
3. Members are asked to identify the insects in the picture.
4. Members may color the picture and draw other insects that were pests in their home states.

Group Discussion:

Members share their pictures and identify the insects in the picture, starting at upper left: grasshopper, bedbug, mosquito, cockroach and boll weevil. The leader asks members to share experiences they have had with insect pests. Stories may include farming or gardening problems or insects that are not included in the picture. Members' recollections may vary depending on where they grew up or worked.

Members share their sentences about something that annoys them. The leader asks for suggestions about how to cope with the various annoyances mentioned. The leader points out that some things can be changed and some things cannot be changed. If things can be changed, communicating about the problem may help. If the annoyance cannot be changed, ideas for coping may include distracting oneself, avoiding the irritating person or situation, and practicing positive thinking. Sharing feelings and ideas for coping strategies instills hope and a feeling of community.

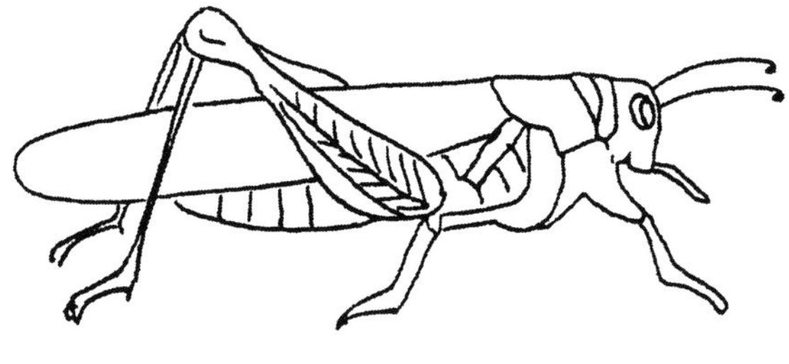

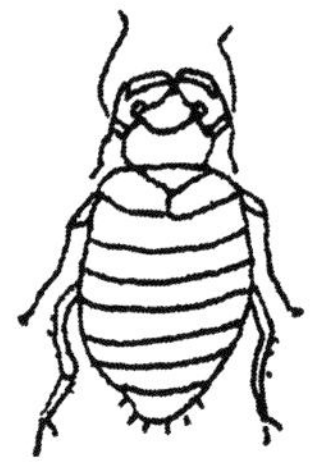

Something that bugs me:

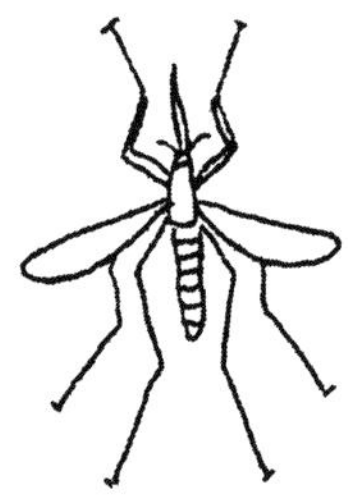

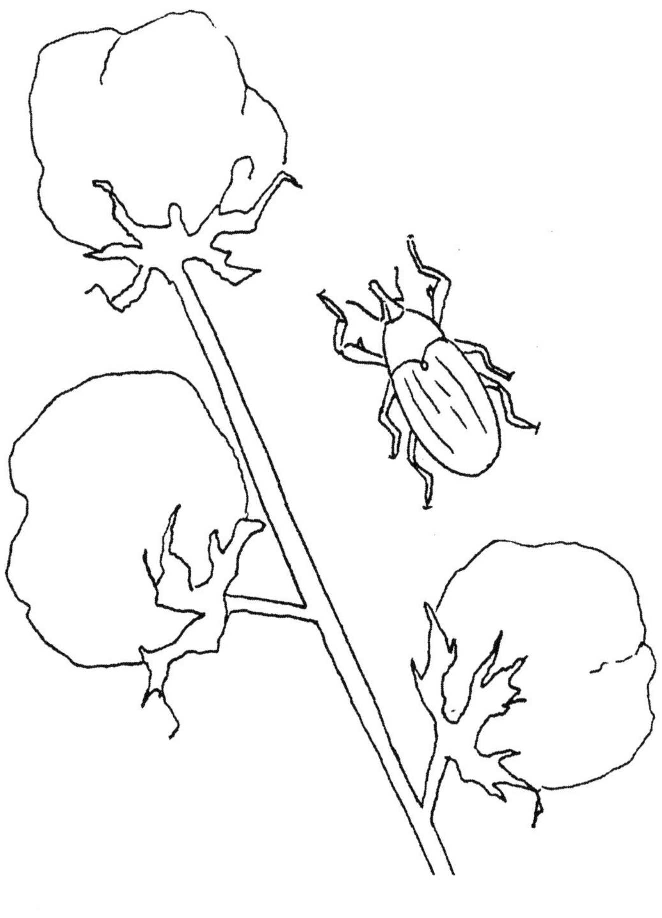

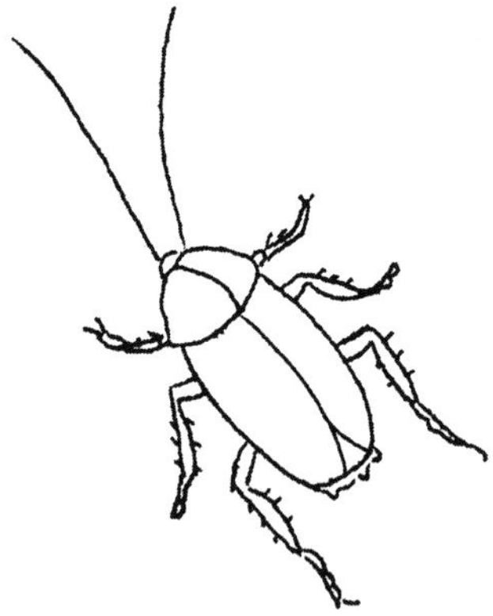

Exercise 4

DINNER TIME

Purpose:

- Share family backgrounds to increase understanding of self and others.
- Share feelings about the common experience of dinner to increase relatedness and enhance coping skills.

Materials:

One photocopy of the illustration for each group member; pencils, crayons, or fine-line colored felt pens.

Procedure:

1. Materials are passed out and members are asked to identify the picture.
2. Members are asked to think about memories of family dinners.
3. The sentences are read aloud and members are asked to fill in the blanks.
4. Members are encouraged to draw family members around the table in the empty chairs. Members may color the picture.

Group Discussion:

Members share their pictures and sentences. Some members may remember eating around a round oak table similar to the one in the picture. The leader asks members how they felt about dinner with their families, and whether the experience was pleasant or unpleasant. Sharing family backgrounds helps to build feelings of community.

Members share their sentences about things they like and don't like about dinner now. If dissatisfactions are expressed, the leader asks for suggestions to help members cope more effectively with frustrations. Suggestions might include communicating with table mates, asking for different seating arrangements, or talking to dietary personnel about problems. Sharing ideas for coping reduces frustration and feelings of helplessness.

Dinner Time

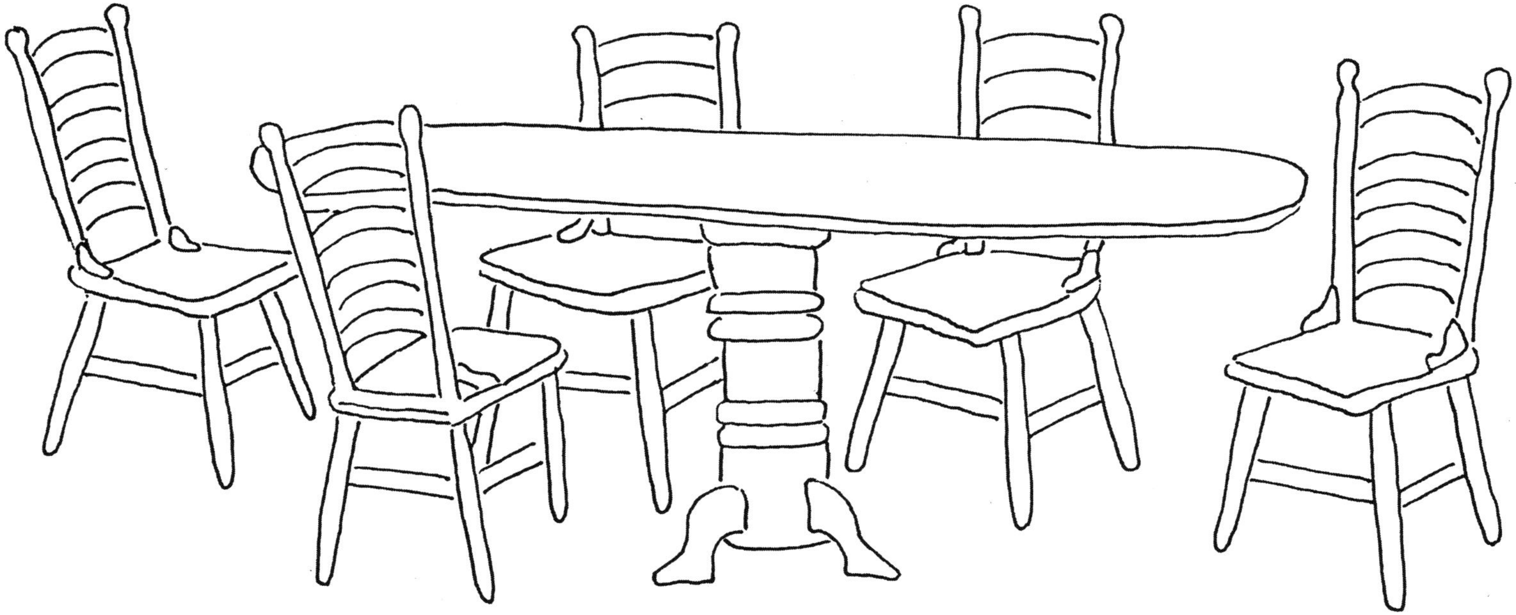

Something I recall about family dinners: ______________________________

____

Something I like about dinner now: ______________________________

____

Something I don't like about dinner now: ______________________________

____

Exercise 5

ABSENCE MAKES THE HEART GROW FONDER

Purpose:

- Encourage expression of feelings in a supportive group setting.
- Raise awareness of the feelings of others to promote group cohesion.

Materials:

One photocopy of the illustration for each group member; pencils, crayons, or fine-line colored felt pens.

Procedure:

1. Materials are distributed and the caption is read aloud.
2. Members are asked what the saying could mean.
3. The sentence fragments are read aloud and members are asked to fill in the blanks.
4. Members who wish may color the picture or add drawings to the illustration.

Group Discussion:

The leader points out that absence does not always make the heart grow fonder. Members share their sentences telling whether the saying was true for them or not and how they felt about those relationships. Members may recall being separated from family members, friends, or loved ones who served in the armed forces or had to move away for other reasons. The leader asks members to tell how they coped with these difficult circumstances. Many members may currently be separated from loved ones. The leader asks members for ideas about how to stay in touch. Sharing coping techniques helps to reduce isolation.

The leader asks if anyone can identify the forget-me-not flowers in the picture and tell what color the flowers usually are. Members are asked to tell any memories they have related to seeing the flowers growing in their home state or planting them in their gardens. Sharing about a common subject increases group cohesion.

Absence Makes the Heart Grow Fonder

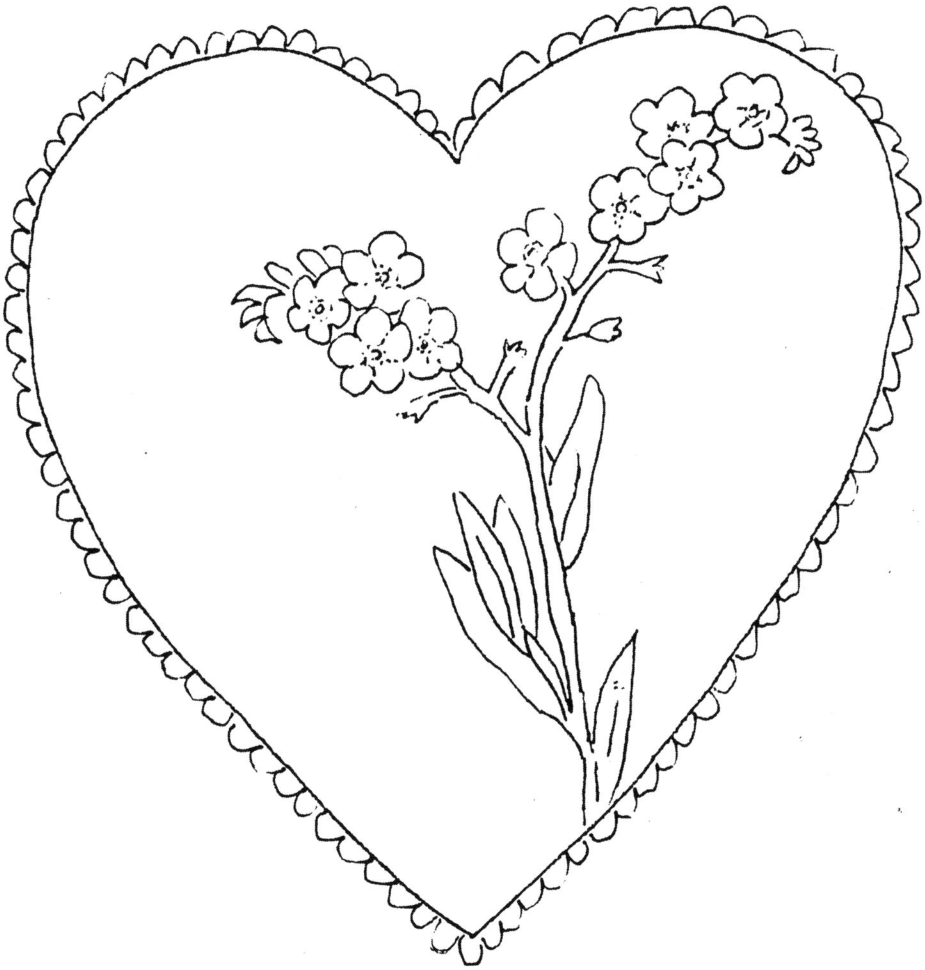

I found this saying to be true because: ____________________

____

I did not find this saying to be true because: ______________

____

Exercise 6

LET'S PATCH THINGS UP

Purpose:

- Open up feelings about unresolved conflicts.
- Share ideas about how to resolve conflicts with others.

Materials:

One photocopy of the illustration for each group member; pencils, crayons, or fine-line colored felt pens.

Procedure:

1. Materials are distributed and members are asked to tell what the woman in the illustration is doing.
2. The sentences are read aloud and members are asked what the saying "Let's patch things up" could mean.
3. Members who write are encouraged to complete the sentence at the bottom of the picture.
4. Members may color the illustration if they wish and draw in a patchwork quilt design they remember on the picture of the blanket.

Group Discussion:

Members share their illustrations and sentences. The leader asks how members feel about unresolved conflicts. Members are asked to give ideas about how to resolve conflicts. The leader demonstrates respect for members' feelings. If a member tells about a conflict with someone who is deceased, that member is asked to tell what they would like to say to the person if they could talk to them.

Exploring feelings about conflict helps members to work through unresolved issues and develop new ways to cope with interpersonal problems.

Members are encouraged to share memories about patchwork quilts and quilting bees. Members may recall popular quilt patterns, such as the Wedding Ring, Sunbonnet Sue, or Dutch Girl designs. Members can also be asked about the woman's sweater in the illustration. Some members may recognize the cable stitch and be able to tell about their own experiences knitting or crocheting.

Sharing about a common subject builds feelings of belonging.

Let's Patch Things Up

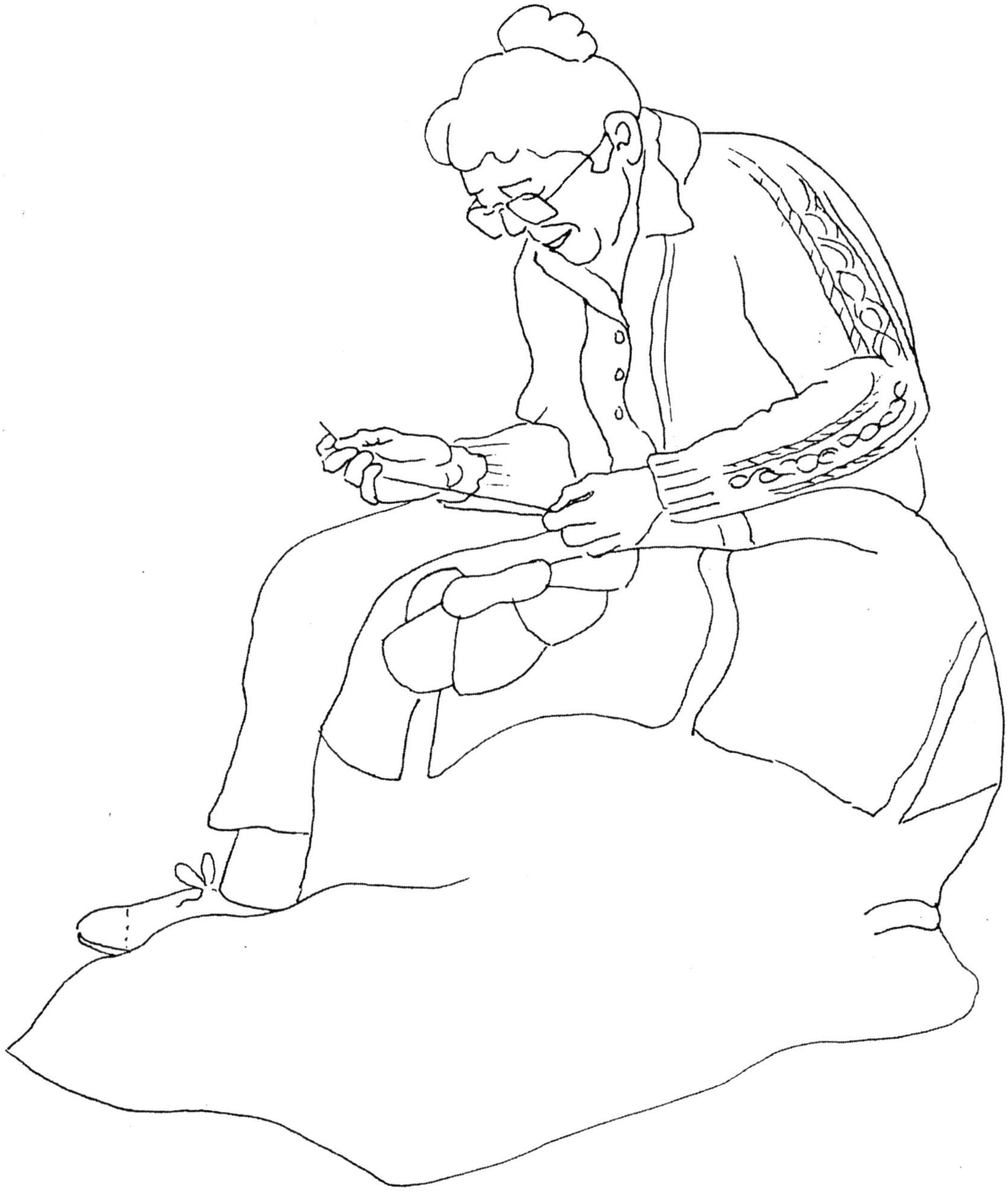

I'd like to patch things up with: ______________________

Exercise 7

FAVORITE WISHES

Purpose:

- Explore unmet needs and frustrations to increase understanding of self and others.
- Share ideas for coping with unfulfilled wishes.

Materials:

One photocopy of the illustration for each group member; pencils, crayons, or fine-line colored felt pens.

Procedure:

1. While materials are distributed, members are asked to think about favorite wishes they have had.
2. Members are asked to identify the picture and tell whether they have ever made a wish and then blown the fluff off a dandelion to see if the wish would come true.
3. The sentence fragment is read aloud and members who write are asked to fill in the blank with their wish.
4. Members who like may draw pictures they associate with dandelions or wishes and color the picture.

Group Discussion:

Members are asked to share memories about dandelions. Some members may recall eating dandelion greens, drinking dandelion wine, or digging dandelions out of their yard.

Members share their pictures and wishes. The leader points out any common themes that the wishes represent, such as desires for peace, love, or security. Recognizing that wishes often represent universal needs reduces feelings of isolation.

The leader asks for ideas about how to cope with unfulfilled wishes. Ideas might include ways to meet the underlying need expressed by the wish in a different way; for example, the wish may be to visit with a sister in Germany. The need underlying the wish is for companionship. To partially fulfill the need, the member might write to the sister or visit with a friend. Sharing ideas for dealing with unmet needs increases positive coping and feelings of hopefulness.

Favorite Wishes

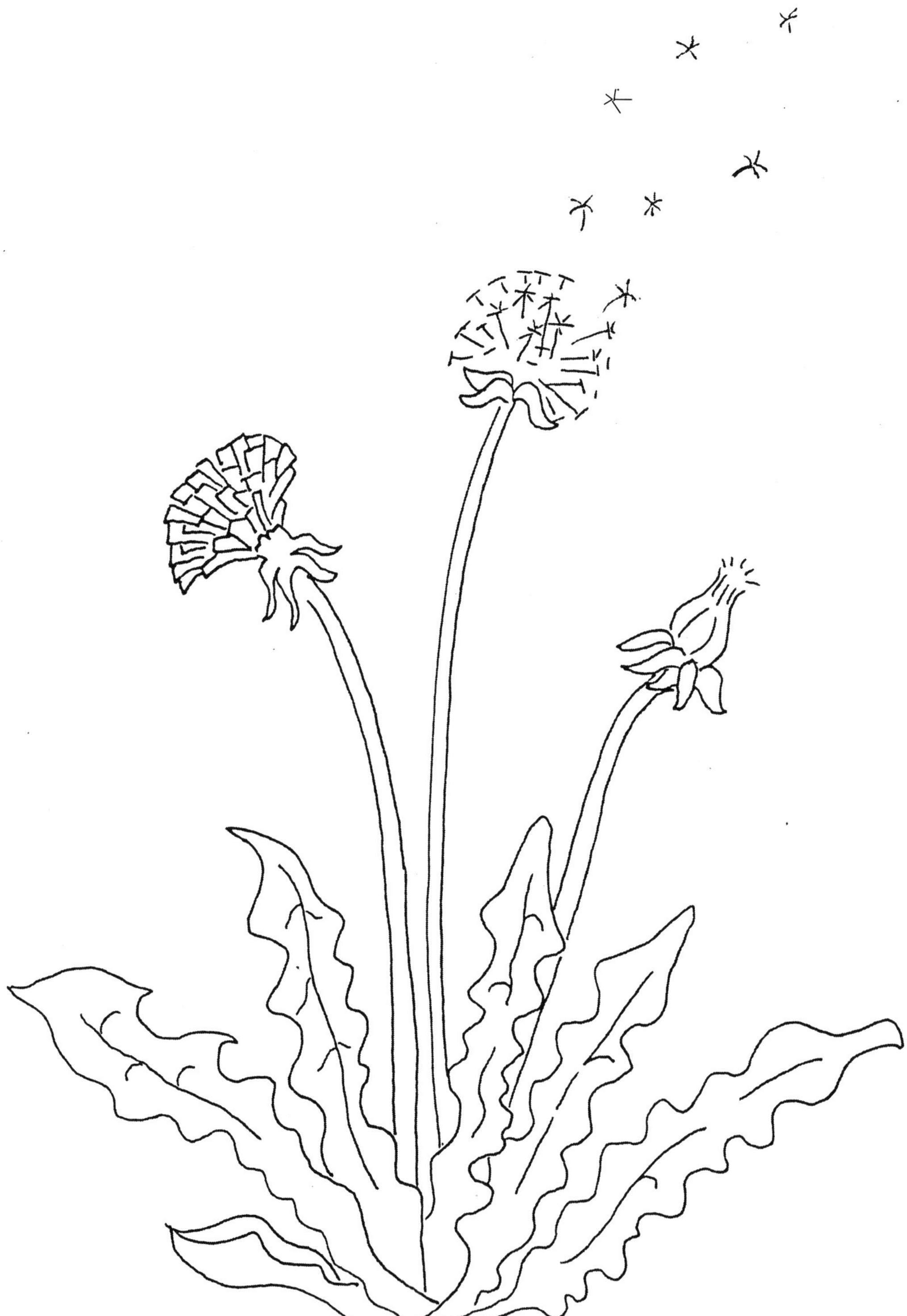

A favorite wish of mine: ______________________________

Exercise 8

GROUCHY AS A BEAR

Purpose:

- Encourage members to express feelings about irritable moods in a supportive group setting.
- Share coping strategies to reduce irritability.

Materials:

One photocopy of the illustration for each group member; pencils, crayons, or fine-line colored felt pens.

Procedure:

1. Materials are passed out and the caption is read aloud.
2. Members are asked to think about times when they feel grouchy and what helps them to feel less irritable.
3. The sentence fragments are read aloud and members who write are asked to fill in the blanks with their ideas.
4. Members who wish may color the bear and draw pictures of things they associate with bears.

Group Discussion:

The leader asks if any member has had an encounter with a hostile, irritable bear in the wild. Members are encouraged to tell about experiences seeing bears, hunting bears, or seeing bears in a zoo. Sharing experiences increases feelings of belonging.

Members share their pictures and sentences about feeling grouchy and how to feel less grouchy. The leader encourages members to think of ways to reduce irritability. Suggestions might include relaxing, eating something, going for a walk, or thinking positive thoughts. The leader points out that everyone feels grouchy at times. Common causes of irritability are fatigue, hunger, pain, and negative thinking. Sharing strategies for coping increases members' ability to handle daily annoyances in a healthy way.

Grouchy as a Bear

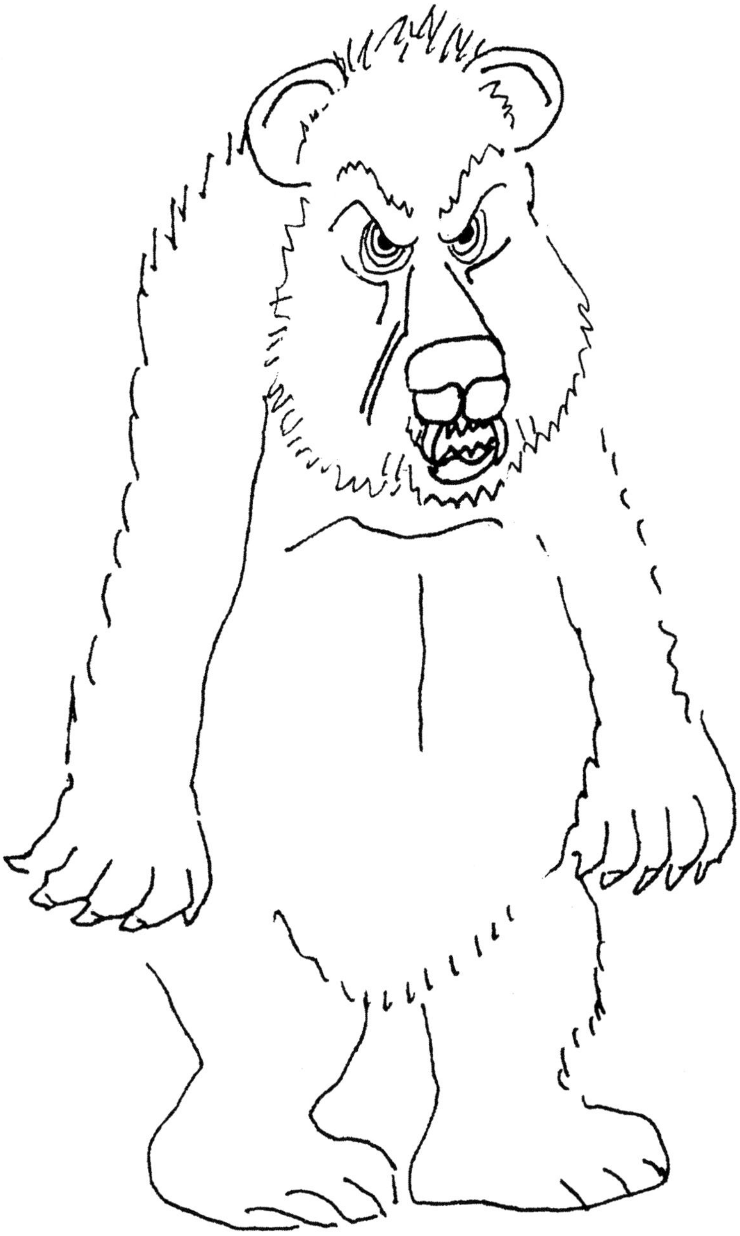

I feel grouchy as a bear when: ______________________________

____

When I feel grouchy it helps to: ____________________________

____

Exercise 9

SINGING A SONG

Purpose:

- Share feelings about music to strengthen identity and sense of self.
- Raise awareness of how to use music to improve one's mood.

Materials:

One photocopy of the illustration for each group member; pencils, crayons, or fine-line colored felt pens.

Procedure:

1. While materials are distributed, members are asked to think about music they like.
2. The sentence fragments are read aloud and members who write are asked to fill in the blanks with a song they would like to sing and a kind of music they enjoy.
3. Members who wish may draw themselves or someone else singing and color the picture.

Group Discussion:

Members share their pictures and sentences. The leader asks if any members have experienced singing for other people. Members are encouraged to share memories about singing and listening to music they enjoy.

The leader points out that music can be used to express emotions and promote relaxation. Members are asked to tell about current opportunities to enjoy music. Ideas might include radio stations or T.V. programs that feature particular types of music. Some members may discover that they have common interests in music with other group members.

Raising members' awareness of interests in common and opportunities for enjoyment reduces self-absorption and promotes feelings of belonging.

Singing a Song

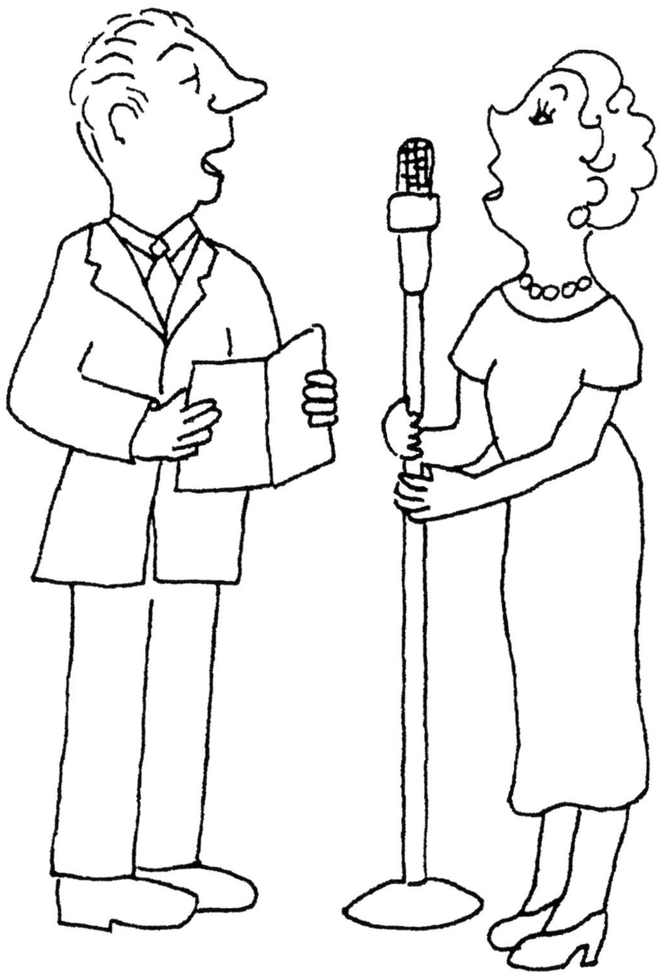

If I had a beautiful singing voice, the song I would like to sing for people is: ________________________________

____

One kind of music I like: ___________________________

____

Exercise 10

HIDING IN A SHELL

Purpose:

- Share feelings to increase understanding of self and others.
- Learn new ways to reduce isolation and withdrawal.

Materials:

One photocopy of the illustration for each group member; pencils, crayons, or fine-line colored felt pens.

Procedure:

1. Materials are passed out and members are asked to tell what the saying "Hiding in a shell" could mean.
2. The sentence fragments are read aloud and members who write are asked to note down times when they feel like crawling in a shell and things that help them to come out of their shell.
3. Members who wish may color the picture or draw something they associate with the illustration of the chicken and the egg.

Group Discussion:

Members share their pictures and memories associated with chickens and eggs. Some members may have raised chickens, gathered eggs, or seen a baby chick come out of its shell.

The leader explains that "Hiding in a shell" can mean to withdraw from other people. A person might want to hide in a shell when they feel frightened or insecure or wish to avoid another person for some reason. Members are asked to tell about times when they feel like hiding in a shell.

The leader asks members to tell about something that helps them to come out of their shell. Ideas might include curiosity, friendly attitudes, or a desire to be included in a pleasant activity. Talking about decisions to participate or withdraw raises members' awareness of how choices about interacting affect a person's mood and self-esteem.

Hiding in a Shell

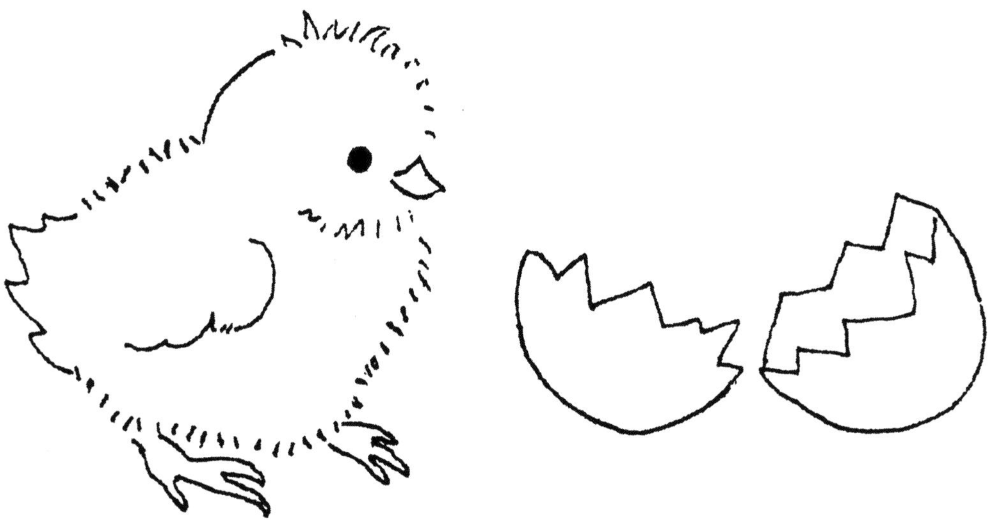

I feel like crawling back in my shell when: ________________

____

Something that helps me to come out of my shell and feel good about myself: ______________________________

____

____

Exercise 11

FAMILY FUN

Purpose:

- Build feelings of belonging by sharing family background information.
- Practice recalling pleasant activities to gain perspective on past events.

Materials:

One photocopy of the illustration for each group member; pencils, crayons, or fine-line colored felt pens. ***Optional:*** Popcorn snack if diet considerations are not an issue.

Procedure:

1. Materials are distributed and the leader asks members to identify the picture.
2. The sentence fragment is read aloud and members are asked to fill in the blank.
3. Members who wish may color the picture and add items associated with popcorn or other family activities that were fun.

Group Discussion:

Members share their pictures and memories about popping corn or other family activities that were enjoyable. Memories might include popping corn in a fireplace or over an open campfire. Some members may have made popcorn balls or enjoyed popcorn at the movies. Sharing pleasant memories that others may have in common helps to reduce isolation and build group cohesion.

The leader points out that sometimes memories become weighted on the negative side, especially if a person is depressed or has suffered a loss or tragedy. Remembering happy times as well as sad times helps to add perspective to the meaning of life.

Family Fun

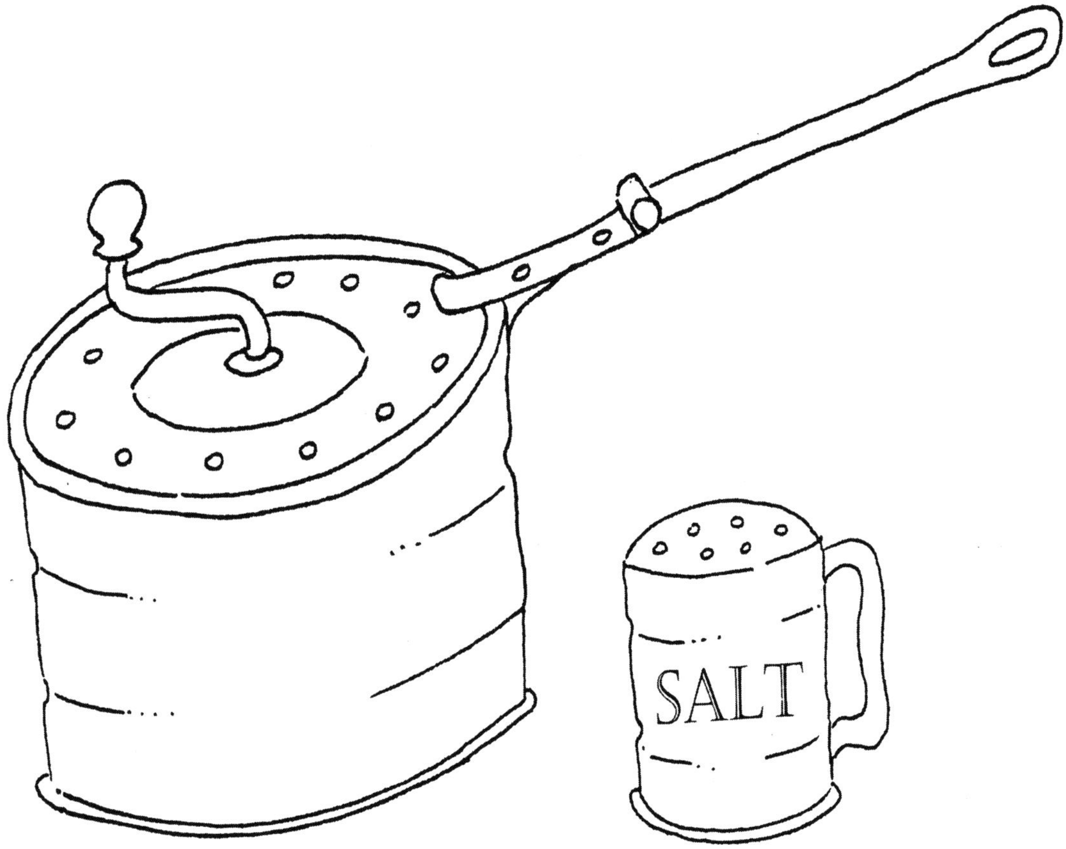

Something we enjoyed doing together as a family: _____

____

____

____

Exercise 12

IRON OUT THE WRINKLES

Purpose:

- Reminiscence about common past experiences to increase relatedness.
- Share feelings and ideas for coping to reduce frustration.

Materials:

A photocopy of the illustration for each group member; pencils, crayons, or fine-line colored felt pens.

Procedure:

1. Materials are distributed and the caption is read aloud.
2. Group members are asked to think about what the saying "Iron out the wrinkles" could mean.
3. The sentence fragments are read aloud and members are asked to fill in the blanks.
4. Members who wish may color the picture and create designs on the fabric in the illustration of something they have ironed or seen someone else iron.

Group Discussion:

The group leader asks members to tell what "Iron out the wrinkles" could mean. Some members may suggest concrete answers about ironing clothes and other members may suggest that the saying refers to solving problems. The leader acknowledges and shows appreciation for all the responses. The leader asks if anyone can think of an example from their own life of solving a problem by "Ironing out the wrinkles." Problem solving might include defining the problem, taking some action, or asking for help.

Group members are asked to share their pictures and sentences. Members may recall the days before permanent press clothing when everything was ironed. The leader asks members to share feelings about care of their clothes. If frustrations are expressed, members are asked to tell how they cope with problems. Ideas might include communicating with laundry personnel, marking personal items, or hand washing if this is possible. Sharing feelings and ideas for coping reduces frustration and isolation.

Iron Out the Wrinkles

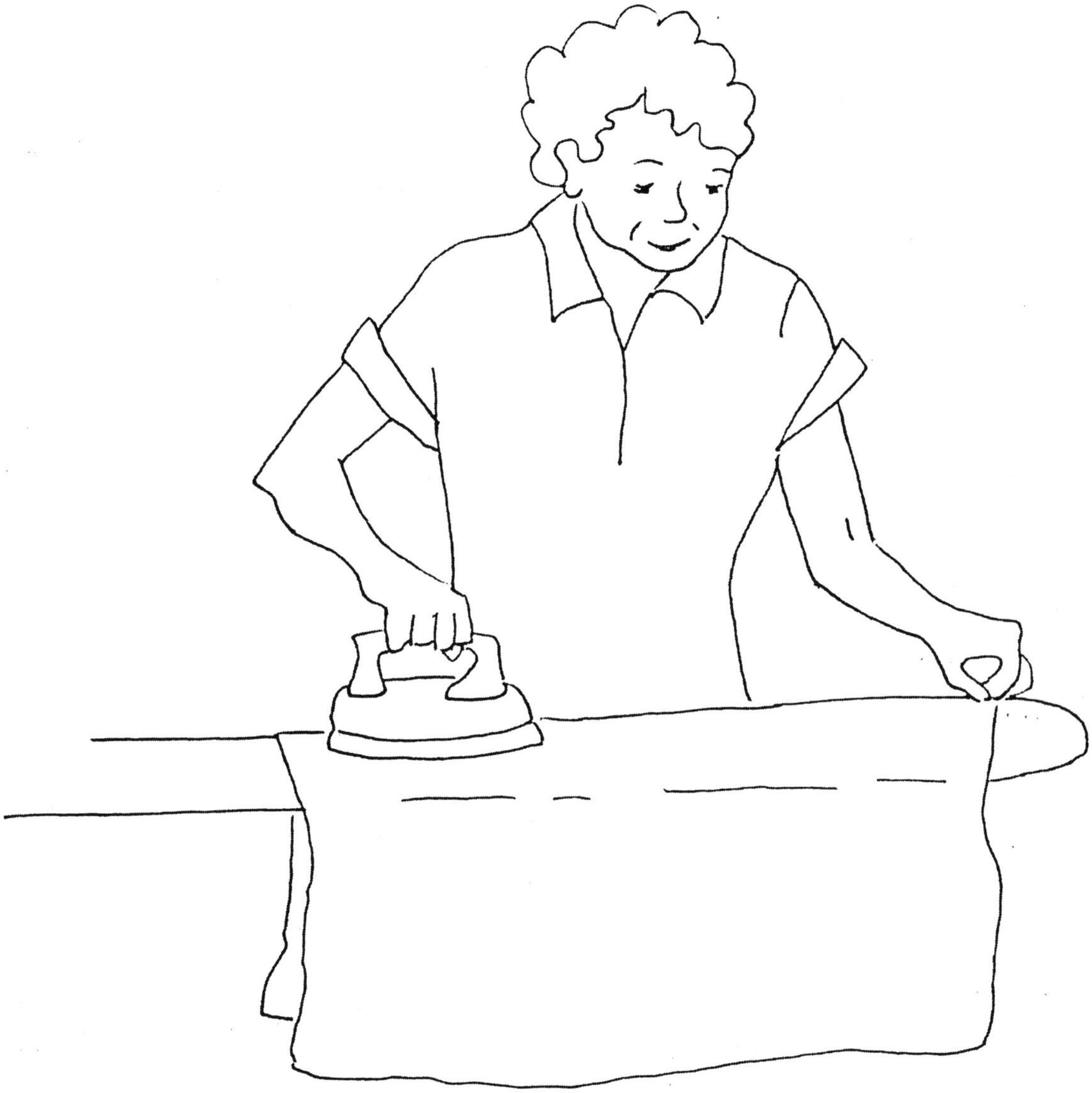

How ironing was done when I was a child: ____________

____

____

How I feel about the care of my clothes now: ____________

____

____

Exercise 13

IF MY MOOD WAS A COLOR

Purpose:

- Practice talking about feelings in a group setting.
- Increase awareness about how a person can improve their mood.

Materials:

One photocopy of the illustration for each group member; pencils, crayons, or fine-line colored felt pens.

Procedure:

1. Each member is given a photocopy of the illustration, a pencil, crayons, or felt pens.
2. Members are asked to think about how different colors can represent different moods.
3. The sentence fragments are read aloud and members who write are asked to fill in the blanks with ideas about their moods.
4. From the crayons given them, members are asked to choose colors to represent their mood and draw a picture in the frame that depicts their mood.

Group Discussion:

Members are asked to share their sentences and pictures, explaining how the color and picture represent their mood. The leader explains that people do not always have the same feelings about colors; for example, red might represent excitement to one person and anger to another person. This exercise encourages members to express their feelings and show acceptance for the feelings of others.

Members are asked to share personal experiences about drawing or painting. The leader points out that producing art is helpful to some people in expressing feelings and coping with emotions. Members are asked to share ideas about current opportunities to participate in arts and crafts. Raising awareness about how to use art as a coping strategy may increase members' ability to deal effectively with emotions.

If My Mood Was a Color

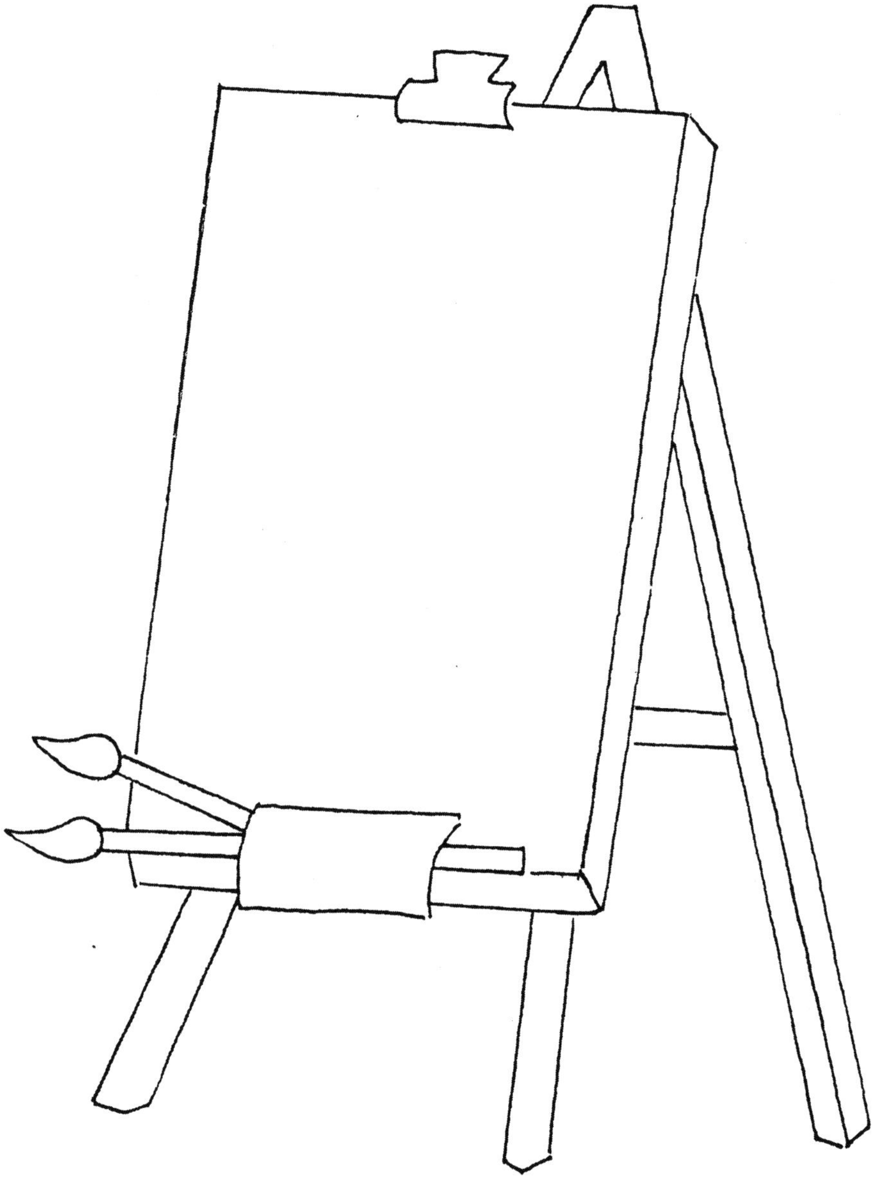

Today I feel: ____

If my mood was a color, it would be: __________________

One way I could improve my mood is to: ____________

____

Exercise 14

SHARING GOOD TIMES

Purpose:

- Build feelings of belonging by sharing about a nonthreatening subject.
- Increase positive focus on past and present experiences.

Materials:

One photocopy of the illustration for each group member; pencils, crayons, or fine-line colored felt pens.

Procedure:

1. Materials are distributed and the leader asks members to identify the picture.
2. The sentence fragment is read aloud and members who can write are asked to fill in the blanks with a memory about ice cream.
3. Members who wish may draw pictures associated with their memories of ice cream, such as ice cream cones or sundaes.

Group Discussion:

Members show their pictures and share memories about making or eating ice cream. The leader may ask questions to help stimulate memories, such as, where the salt was used and which flavors or fruits were added to the ice cream. Some members may recall making "snow ice cream" in the winter by mixing cream and sugar with snow.

The leader then asks members about current opportunities to enjoy a pleasant treat. Members may get ideas from each other about how to increase their enjoyment of snacks. The leader points out that healthful food substitutes are becoming more available such as sugar free or fat free frozen desserts.

Sharing pleasant memories and ideas for coping increases a sense of hope and belonging.

Sharing Good Times

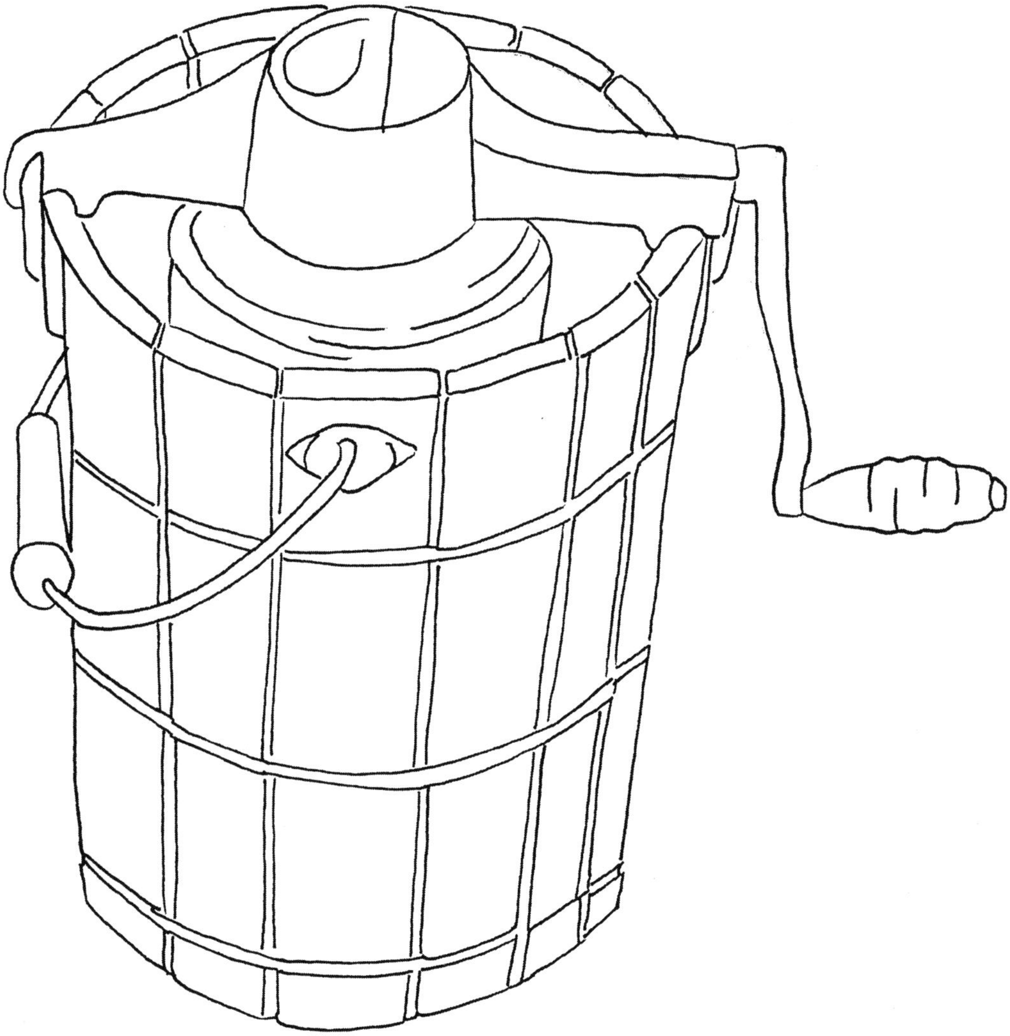

A memory I have of making or eating ice cream: ________

____

____

Exercise 15

AN IRISH BLESSING

Purpose:

- Practice sharing feelings of goodwill to promote self-esteem and interest in others.
- Share memories about a nonthreatening subject to promote relatedness and a sense of belonging.

Materials:

One photocopy of the illustration for each group member; pencils, crayons, or fine-line colored felt pens.

Procedure:

1. Materials are distributed and the Irish blessing is read aloud.
2. Members are asked to think about the meaning of the lines in the blessing and what they would include if they wrote an Irish blessing.
3. Members are asked to fill in the blank with something they would wish for someone. Ideas might include Luck, Health, Happiness, Comfort, Peace, or other good wishes.
4. Members may color the picture, fold the handout into fourths to form a card, and sign the inside of the card.

Group Discussion:

Members share their ideas about what they think is important to wish for others and why they chose a particular wish. The leader explains that the origin of Irish Blessings is unclear, but the intent of the blessings is to promote feelings of warmth, love, comfort, and good fortune. The Irish had a difficult history, but in Irish Blessings they tried to stay positive and wish good fortune to others. The leader points out that focusing on positive wishes for others often lifts ones mood. Members may exchange their cards with other group members or choose to give their cards to someone outside the group.

The leader asks if any group members are Irish or if anyone has a story to tell about St. Patrick's Day or Ireland. Sharing positive personal information increases feelings of belonging.

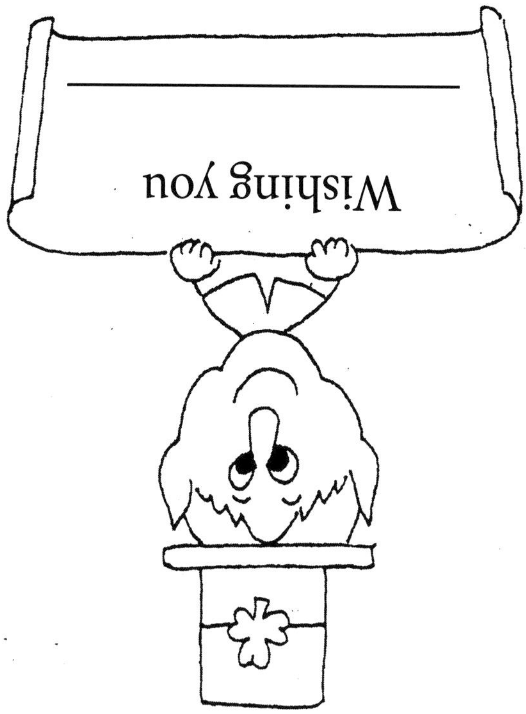

An Irish Blessing

May soft be the grass you walk on,

May fair be the skies above you,

May true be the joys that surround you,

May dear be the hearts that love you.

Exercise 16

LONELY LITTLE PETUNIA

Purpose:

- Share feelings about loneliness and isolation.
- Gain new perspectives on coping with isolation and estrangement.

Materials:

A photocopy of the illustration for each group member; pencils, crayons or fine-line colored felt pens. ***Optional:*** Recording of the song "Lonely Little Petunia (In an Onion Patch).

Procedure:

1. While materials are distributed, members are asked to think about times in their lives when they felt lonely and different than other people.
2. Members are asked to identify the flower in the picture and read the sentence fragment.
3. Members are asked to fill in the blanks and may color the picture if they wish.
4. If available, the song "Lonely Little Petunia (In An Onion Patch)" is played.

Group Discussion:

Members are asked to share memories about petunias or other flowers they have grown, or flowers that bloomed where they grew up. Members may recall having gardens or house plants that they can describe to the group. Sharing interests helps to promote relatedness.

Members are asked to share any memories they have of the song "Lonely Little Petunia (In An Onion Patch)." The leader asks members to talk about the meaning of the song's title "Lonely Little Petunia (In An Onion Patch)." Members share their pictures and tell about times when they felt lonely or estranged from others and how they coped with these feelings. Sharing ideas about coping skills helps to strengthen techniques for dealing with stress.

I feel like a lonely petunia in an onion patch when: ____

____

____

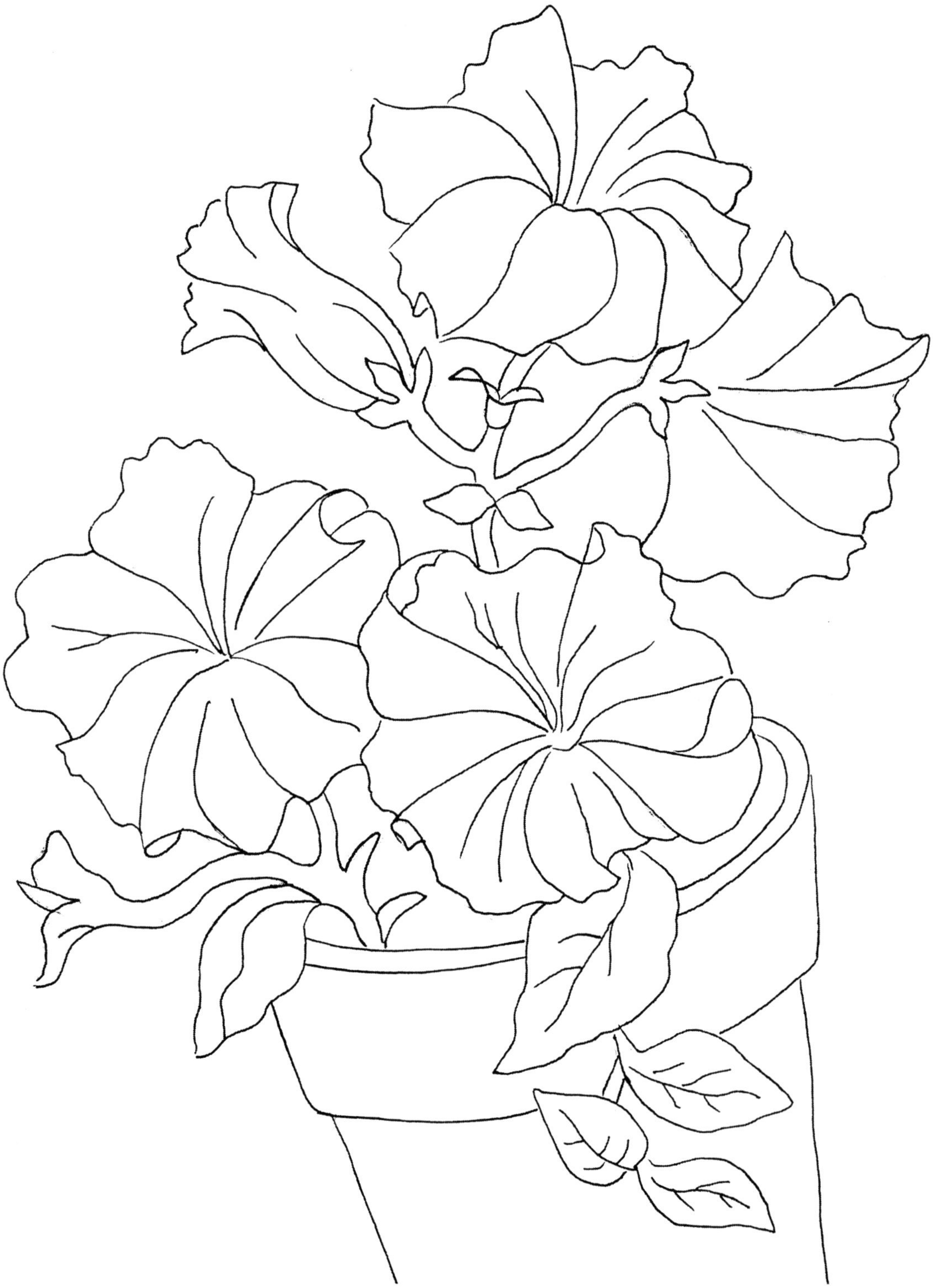

Exercise 17

LET IT SNOW

Purpose:

- Share memories about a nonthreatening topic to increase relatedness.
- Gain insight about coping with adversity to instill hope.

Materials:

One photocopy of the illustration for each group member; pencils, crayons or fine-line colored felt pens. ***Optional:*** A recording of the song, "Let it Snow! Let it Snow! Let it Snow!"

Procedure:

1. Materials are passed out and the caption is read aloud.
2. The sentence fragments are read aloud and members are asked to fill in the blanks.
3. Members who wish may draw snow-related pictures and color the illustration.
4. If available, the song "Let it Snow! Let it Snow! Let it Snow!" is played.

Group Discussion:

Members share their pictures and tell about memories they have about snow. Some members may recall sleigh riding, shoveling snow, building snow men, or playing games in the snow such as Fox and Goose. Sharing about a nonthreatening subject helps to increase trust and promote group cohesion.

Members are asked to recall the lyrics to "Let it Snow! Let it Snow! Let it Snow!" The song not only talks about the weather outside being frightful and not wanting to go out in the storm, but also points out some positives to the situation: a delightful fire, corn to pop, and someone's love to keep them warm. The leader suggests that the song's enduring popularity may be due to the hopeful attitude of focusing on positive things to make hard situations easier to bear. Discussing the benefits of positive thinking raises members' awareness of how positive and negative thoughts affect their moods.

Let It Snow

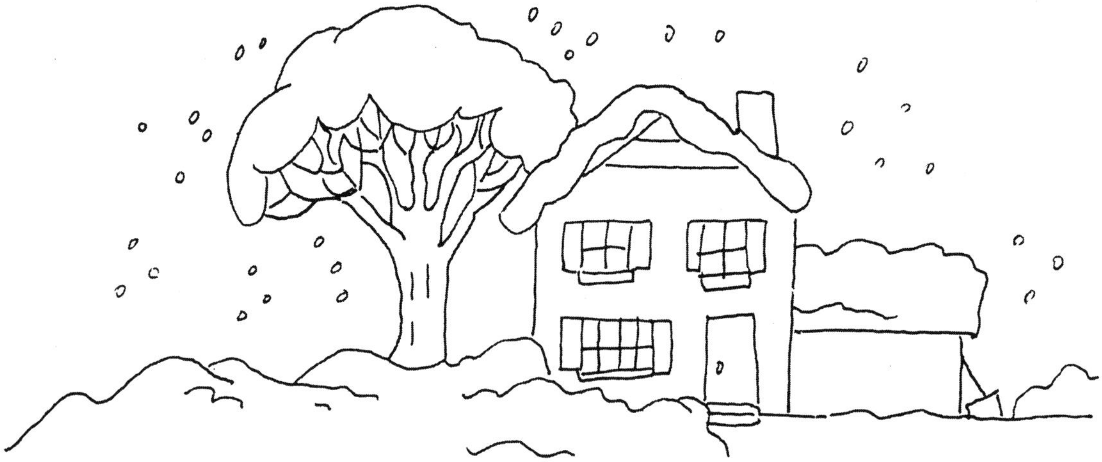

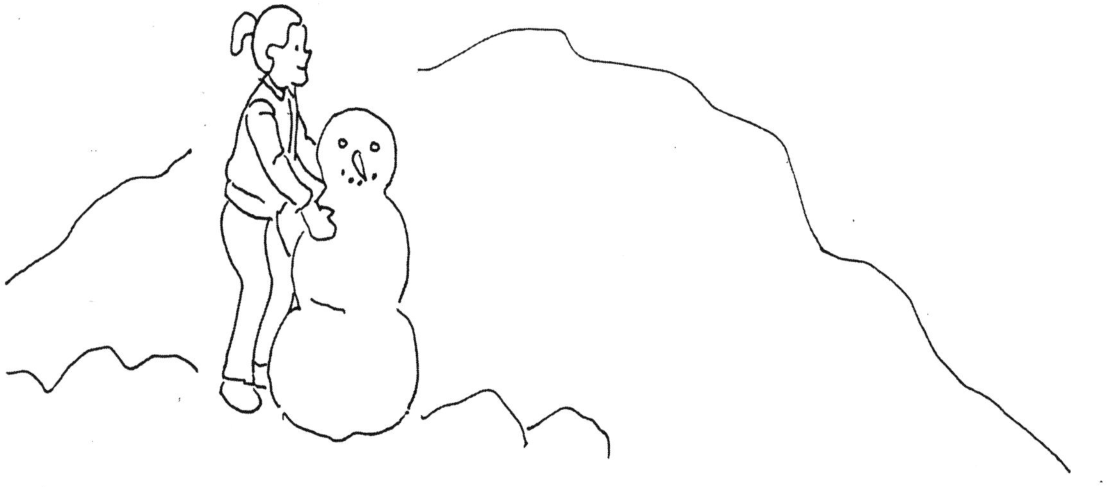

I first saw snow: ______________________________

A memory I have about snow: ____________________

____

____

Exercise 18

PLAYING GAMES

Purpose:

- Share childhood experiences about playing games to build group cohesion and stimulate motivation to participatc in activities.
- Raise awareness of healthy ways to handle difficult interactions with others.

Materials:

One photocopy of the illustration for each group member; pencils, crayons, or fine-line colored felt pens.

Procedure:

1. Materials are passed out and members are asked to identify the game being played in the illustration.
2. Members are asked to think about games they played as children.
3. The sentence fragments are read aloud and members who write are asked to complete the sentences.
4. Members who like to draw may draw a picture of a game they enjoyed. Others may want to color the picture.
5. Members are asked to tell what psychological meanings the phrase "playing games" could have.

Group Discussion:

The leader explains that psychological meanings of the phrase "playing games" might include insincerity, phoniness, or behavior intended to manipulate others. Members are asked to give examples of these kinds of interactions and give ideas of how to react to someone who is "playing games." Ideas might include resisting manipulation, expressing feelings, or ignoring the behavior. Sharing ideas about healthy ways to handle interactions increases coping abilities and reduces feelings of hopelessness.

Members share their sentences and pictures. The leader asks if any members played hopscotch and if they got extra points for picking up small objects. The leader points out that playing games increases interaction and a sense of fun and interest in others. Members are asked to tell about current opportunities to play games or watch games on T.V. Raising awareness of available activities may stimulate interest and motivation to increase participation and reduce feelings of isolation.

Playing Games

A childhood game I enjoyed: ______________________________

A game I enjoy now: ______________________________

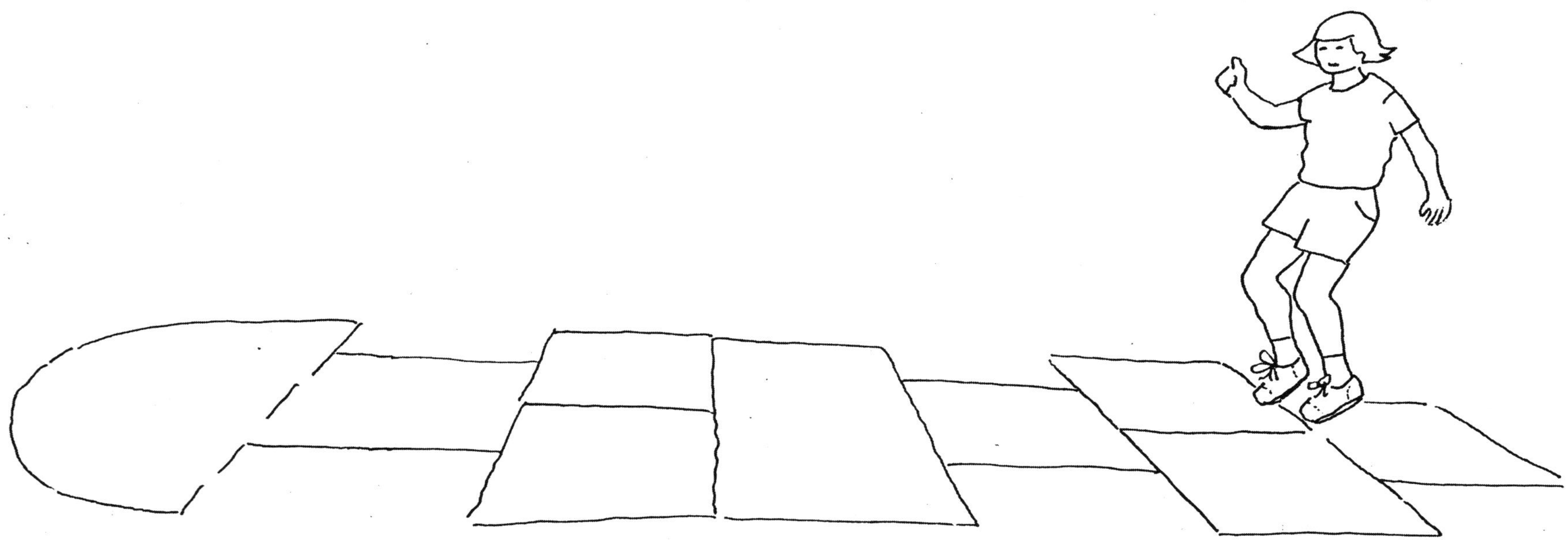

Exercise 19

SOMETIMES I WORRY

Purpose:

- Share feelings of worry and anxiety in a supportive group format.
- Gain insight about ways to reduce worry and anxiety.
- Practice empathy to increase interest in others and reduce self-absorption.

Materials:

One photocopy of the illustration for each group member; pencils, crayons, or fine-line colored felt pens.

Procedure:

1. Materials are distributed and members are asked to think about worries they have.
2. The sentence fragments are read aloud and members are asked to fill in the blanks.
3. Members who wish may color the picture using colors that remind them of worry.

Group Discussion:

Group members share their pictures and sentences. Members are encouraged to express feelings about their worries. The group leader role models empathetic responses, acknowledging that some worries cause feelings of irritation, frustration, or fear. Members are asked if they have similar worries to those expressed by other members. Universality helps to reduce feelings of isolation and despair.

Members share their ideas about how to worry less. Ideas might include communicating about the problem to someone who could help, seeking more information about the problem, or standing up for oneself. The leader points out that there is not a clear cut solution for many things people worry about. When the worry concerns something that cannot be changed, a person can still help themselves to worry less. Ideas include distracting oneself with pleasant activities, practicing meditation, and focusing on positive thoughts. Learning ways to cope with anxiety reduces depression and feelings of hopelessness.

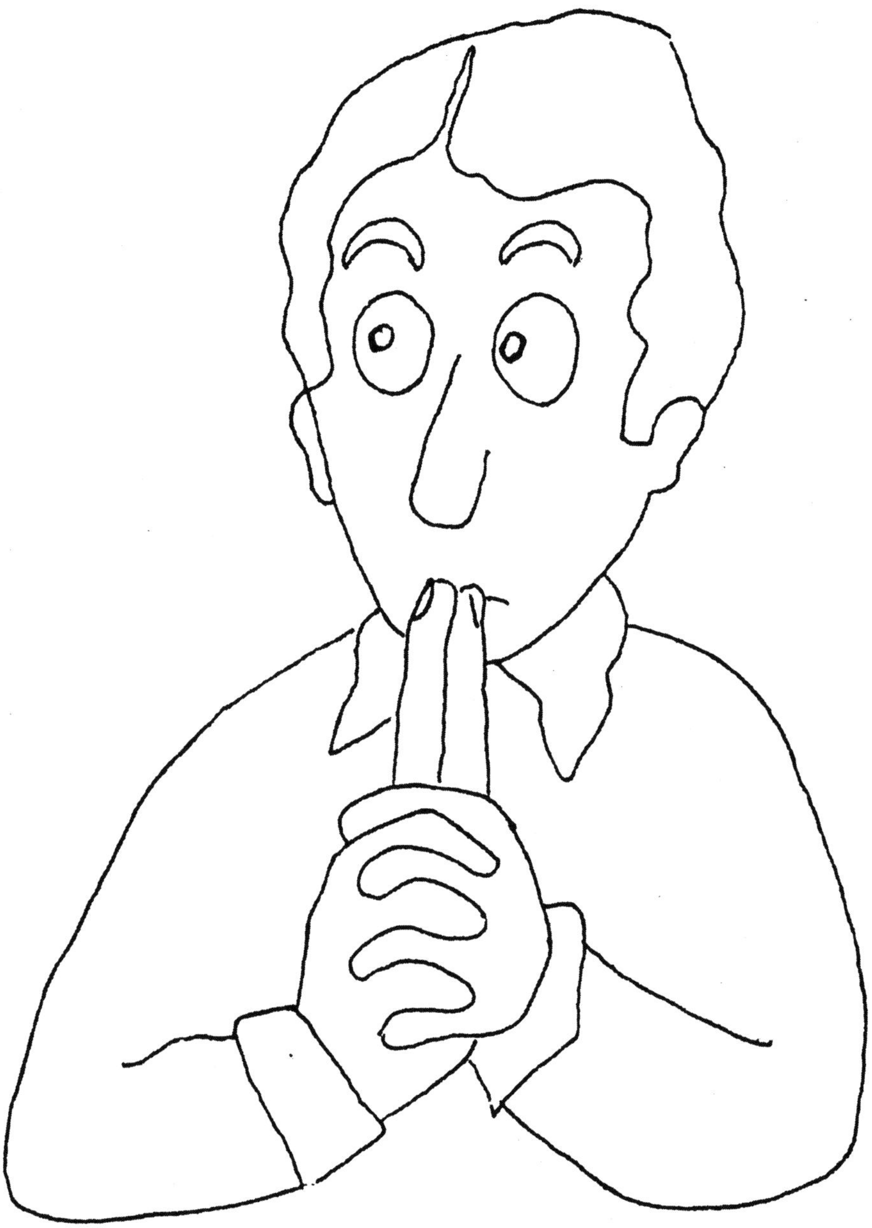

Sometimes I worry about: ______________________________

____

In order to worry less, I could: __________________________

____

Exercise 20

YOU ARE SPECIAL

Purpose:

- Increase sense of identity and self-esteem.
- Share positive personal information in a supportive group setting.

Materials:

One photocopy of the illustration for each group member; pencils, crayons, and fine-line colored felt pens.

Procedure:

1. Materials are distributed and the caption is read aloud.
2. Members are asked to tell what the picture represents.
3. The sentence fragment is read aloud and members who write are asked to fill in the blank.
4. Members who wish may color the picture, draw other constellations, or draw a person looking through the telescope.

Group Discussion:

The leader explains that the purpose of this group discussion is to remind members that each person is unique and special. Members are asked to share their sentences about times when they felt special. Ideas might include getting a first job, having a birthday, or simply going to the beauty shop. The leader points out that everyone likes to feel special and asks members to give ideas about how to help others feel special. Suggestions might include showing appreciation or giving compliments.

This exercise helps to emphasize uniqueness and sense of self which are sometimes diminished in group living situations.

Members are asked to share their pictures and memories about watching the stars and identifying constellations. Sharing about a common experience helps to build group cohesion and a sense of belonging.

You are Special

You are special,
an individual, a masterpiece.
Celebrate your uniqueness.
Don't be someone other than yourself.
Every star is important to the heavens.

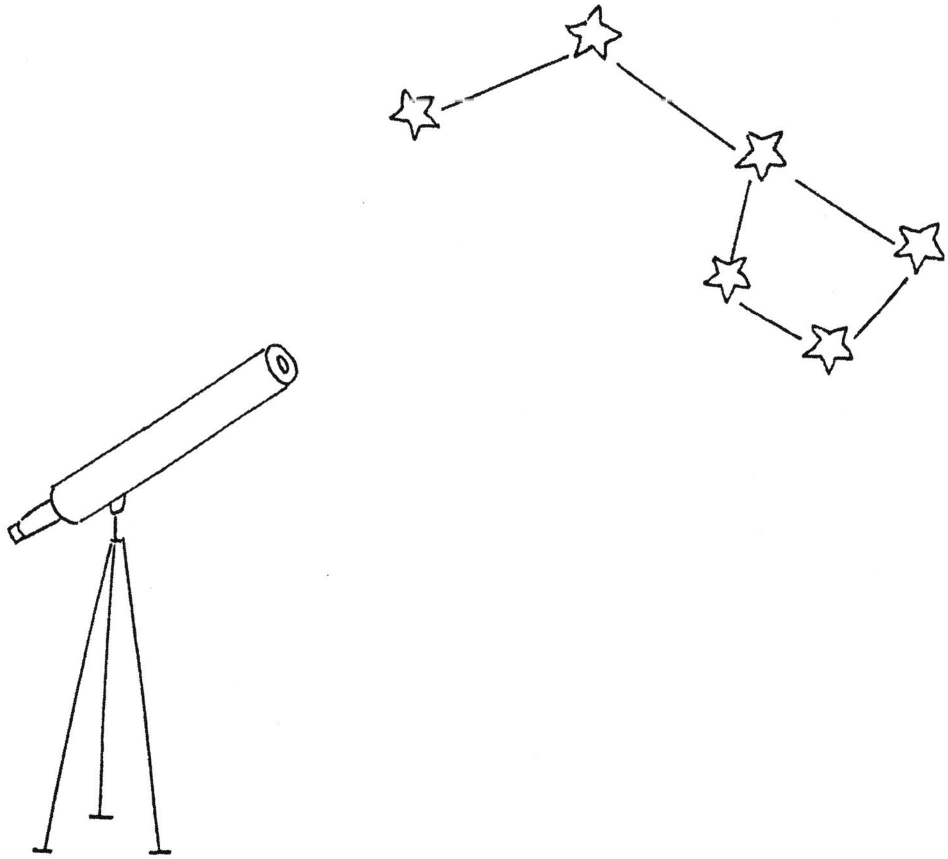

I felt special when: ________________________________

____

Exercise 21

DON'T FENCE ME IN

Purpose:

- Open up feelings of frustration for group support.
- Share ideas for overcoming feelings of isolation and entrapment.

Materials:

One photocopy of the illustration for each group member; pencils, crayons, or fine-line colored felt pens. ***Optional:*** A recording of the song "Don't Fence Me In."

Procedure:

1. Illustrations are passed out and members are asked to identify the picture.
2. Members are asked to think about times when they feel fenced in.
3. Members are asked to complete the sentences and may color the picture and add drawings.
4. If available, a recording of the song "Don't Fence Me In" may be played.

Group Discussion:

If the song has been played, members are asked to share memories about the song or about Roy Rogers, one of the singers who recorded the song. Members who have specific recollections about split rail fences, or building or using other types of fencing, are encouraged to share their experiences to promote bonding and relatedness in the group.

Members share their pictures and sentences about feeling fenced in and tell how they cope with these feelings. The group leader encourages support by acknowledging that everyone has felt fenced in at some time in their lives. Universality reduces feelings of isolation.

Some members may feel fenced in by their current circumstances. Older members often face physical limitations and difficulties with vision and hearing that cause them to feel fenced in. Ideas for coping and feeling less confined are elicited from the group. Sharing frustrations and discussing coping techniques reduces feelings of isolation and helplessness.

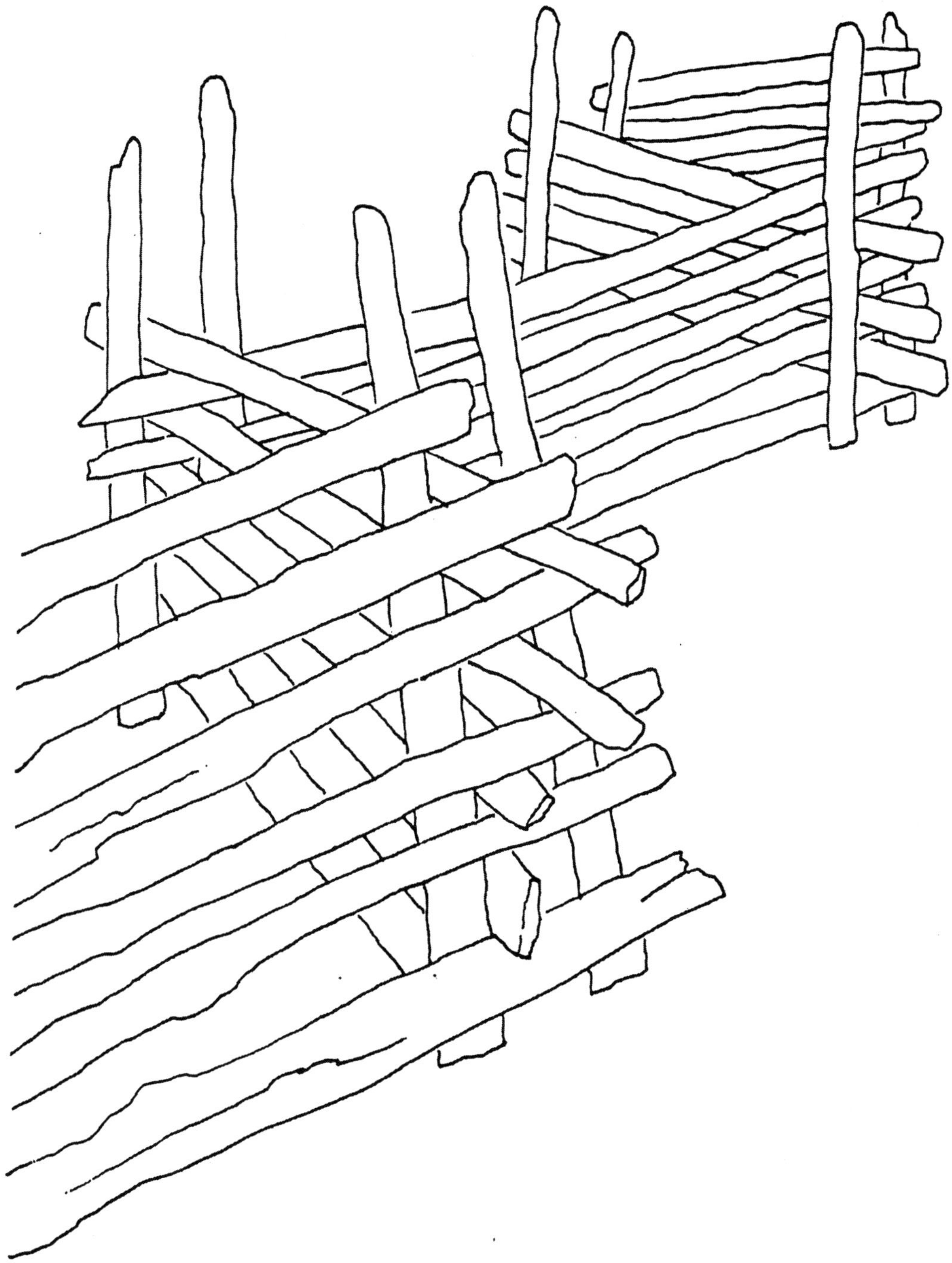

I feel fenced in when: ______________________________

____

Something that helps me to feel less fenced in: _________

____

Exercise 22

A BOUQUET FOR MOTHER

Purpose:

- Share memories about mother to increase trust and relatedness.
- Express feelings through thc usc of drawing and color.

Materials:

One photocopy of the illustration for each group member; pencils, crayons, or fine-line colored felt pens.

Procedure:

1. Materials are passed out and the sentence fragments are read aloud.
2. Members who write are asked to complete the sentences.
3. Members who like to draw are asked to draw and color flowers in the vase that remind them of their mother.
4. Members are asked to draw a likeness of their mother in the picture frame. Members may color the picture if they wish.

Group Discussion:

Members are asked to share their sentences about pleasant memories and wishes regarding mother. Some members may want to share about a mother substitute that was important in their lives. In an older population, many members may have lost their mothers and want to share feelings about this. Sharing feelings builds understanding of others and feelings of relatedness.

Members are asked to share their pictures and tell why they chose particular designs or colors that remind them of their mother. The leader points out that art often helps people to express feelings in a different way. Members are asked to share reminiscence about table cloths, dresser scarves, doilies or other items that can be decorated with handiwork. Emphasizing the value of arts and crafts may increase members interest and involvement in these activities.

A Bouquet for Mother

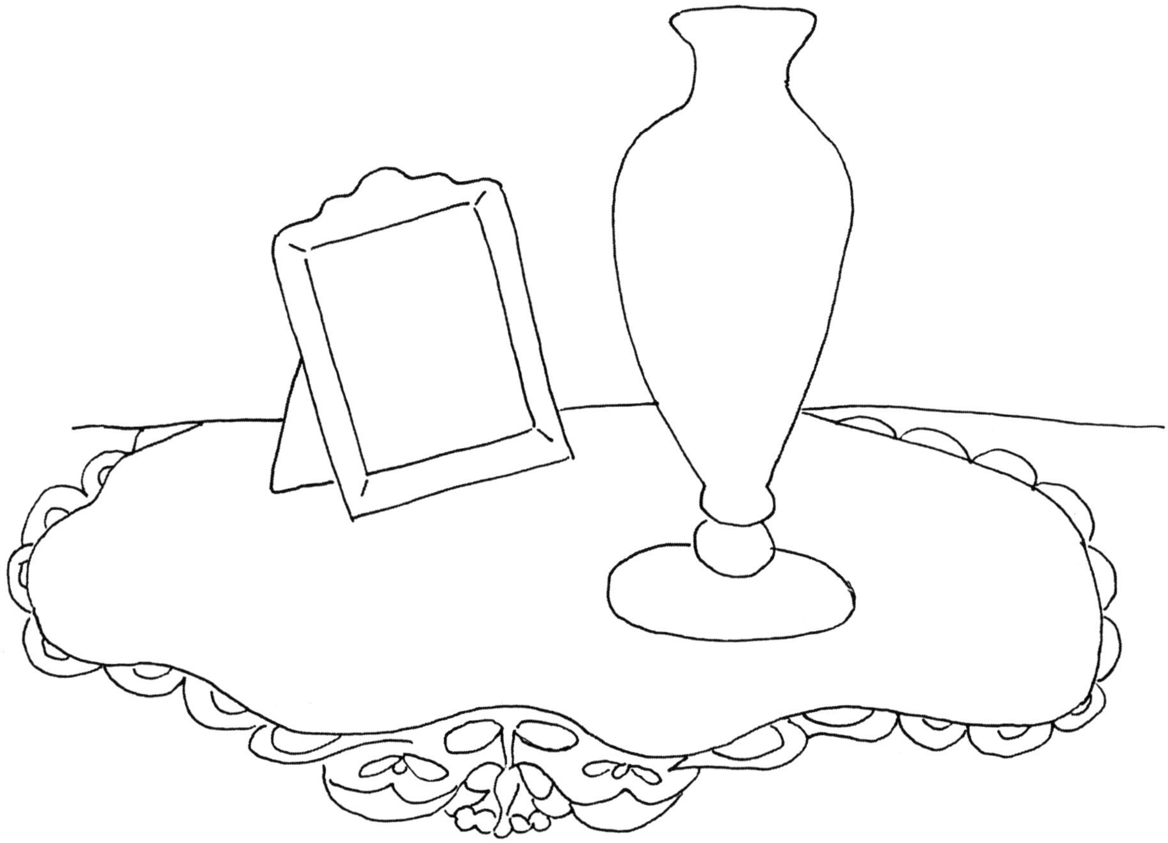

A pleasant memory I have of Mother: ____________________

____

Something I wish I could have done with Mother: ________

____

Exercise 23

GO FLY A KITE

Purpose:

- Encourage reminiscence and ventilation of feelings.
- Provide group ideas and support for effective communication.

Materials:

One copy of the illustration for each group member; pencils, crayons, or fine-line colored felt pens.

Procedure:

1. Materials are distributed and the sentence fragment is read aloud.
2. Members are asked to think about what "Go fly a kite" might mean.
3. Members who write are instructed to complete the sentences.
4. Members who wish may color the picture, draw a tail on the kite, add landscape, or add other kites to the drawing.

Group Discussion:

Members share their memories and pictures about flying kites. Some members may have made kites themselves and have opinions about which kites fly the best. Sharing memories helps to reduce feelings of isolation and stimulates cognitive functioning.

Members are asked to tell what the phrase "Go fly a kite" could mean. The leader explains that it could be an indirect way to tell someone you don't like their ideas or opinions. The group leader asks if anyone has a memory of telling someone to "go fly a kite." Members are asked for ideas on how to express disagreement without starting an argument. Ideas might include acknowledging the other person's right to their opinion while expressing a different point of view on the matter. The leader points out that respecting differences is an important part of building feelings of community.

Go Fly a Kite

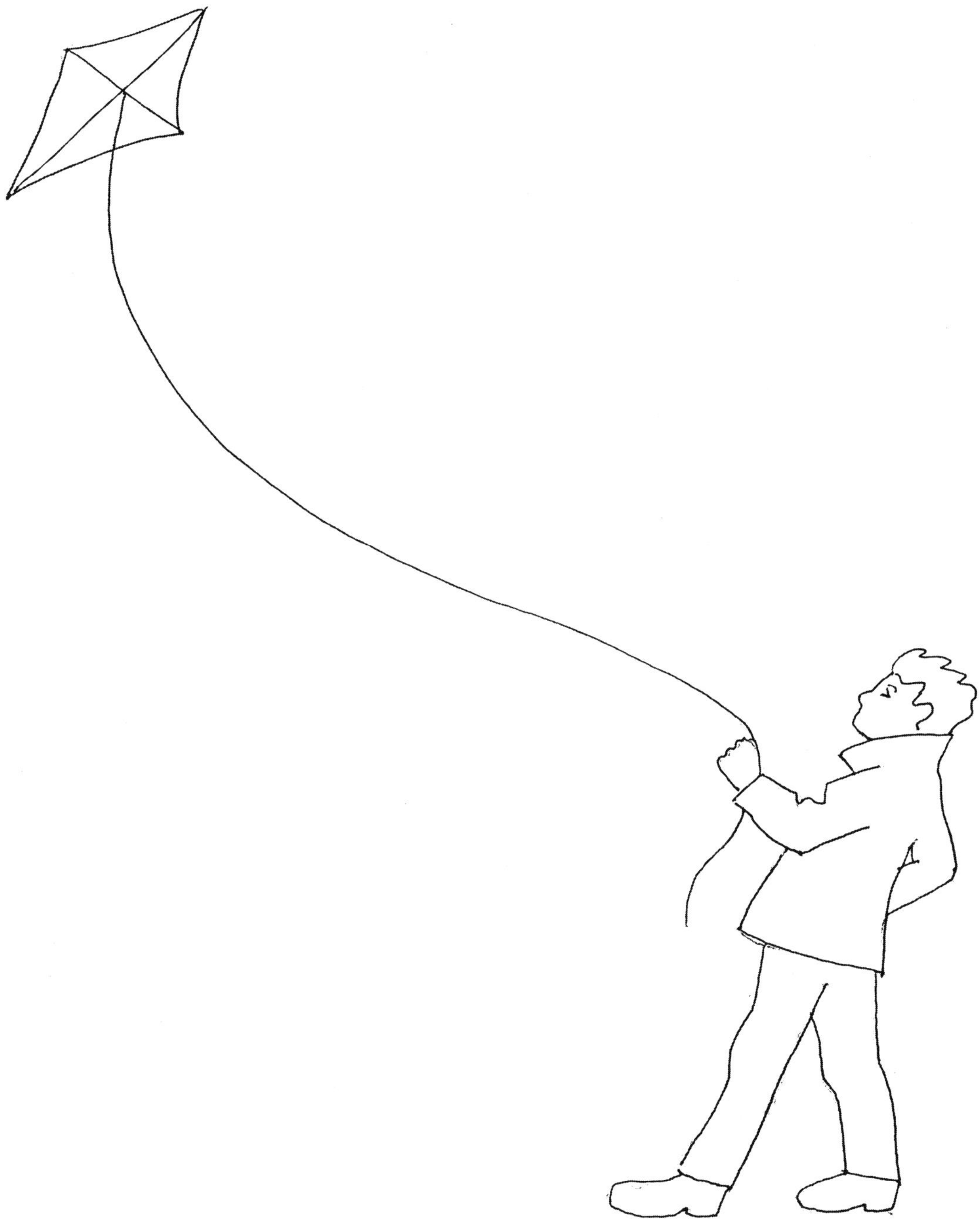

A memory I have about flying kites: ___________________

____

Exercise 24

GROUP ROLES

Purpose:

- Increase members' understanding of their role in group and the roles of others.
- Validate members' feelings to promote group cohesion.

Materials:

One photocopy of the illustration for each group member; pencils, crayons, or fine-line colored felt pens.

Procedure:

1. The leader explains that people play different roles in group and asks members to describe the roles pictured in the illustration.
2. Members are asked to write in the blank a role they have played in group.
3. Members who wish may draw themselves in group and color the illustration.

Group Discussion:

The leader explains that playing different roles in group has advantages and disadvantages. Members are asked to tell how they would feel playing the roles pictured in the illustration and guess how other members might respond to the various roles. The leader helps members to balance the positive and negative aspects of the group roles, such as pointing out that the clown provides humor and entertainment, but may also distract members from dealing with serious issues. Members share their sentences about how they feel in group.

The leader explains that a group member may play different roles in group depending on the topic being discussed or the member's mood. It is important to avoid labeling roles as right or wrong and to encourage better understanding of self and others in group settings.

This exercise helps members to gain insight about how their behavior and the behavior of others effects group process.

Group Roles

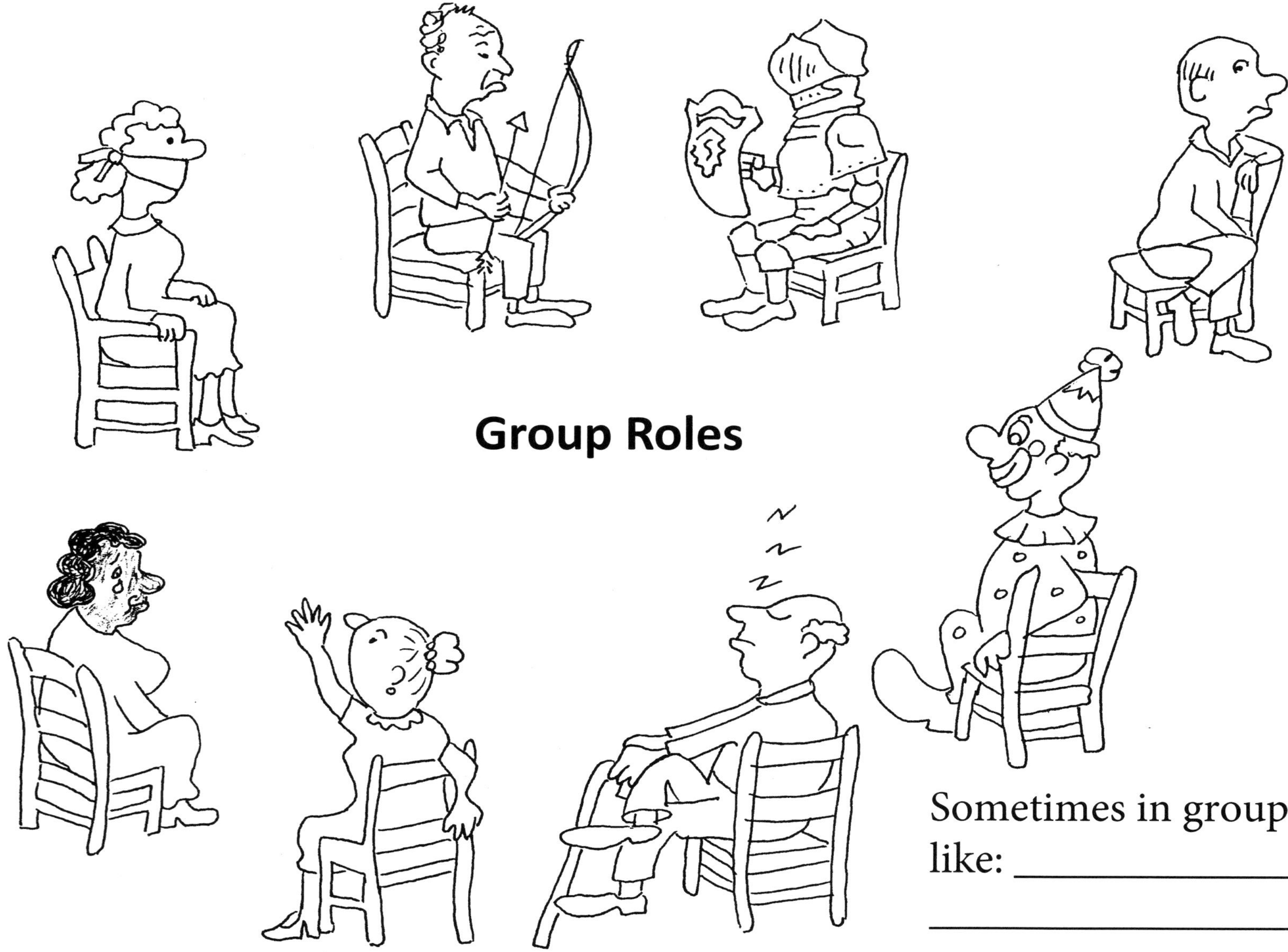

Sometimes in group I feel like: ______________________
____
____

Exercise 25

IF YOU CAN'T TAKE THE HEAT, STAY AWAY FROM THE FIRE

Purpose:

- Increase awareness of self-defeating behavior.
- Learn healthy ways to avoid unnecessary trouble.

Materials:

One photocopy of the illustration for each group member; pencils, crayons, or fine-line colored felt pens.

Procedure:

1. Materials are distributed and the leader reads the caption aloud, "If you can't take the heat, stay away from the fire."
2. Members are asked to tell what they think the saying means.
3. The sentence fragment is read aloud and members who write are asked to fill in the blank with ideas for avoiding trouble.
4. Members who wish may color the picture and draw other items associated with pot bellied stoves, such as shovels and coal buckets.

Group Discussion:

The leader explains that the saying, "If you can't take the heat, stay away from the fire," can mean that a person who wants to avoid problems often needs to stay away from the source of the trouble. Members are asked to share their pictures and ideas. The leader points out that members can't always physically move away from problems, but they can sometimes move their thoughts away from upsetting subjects by relaxing or talking to someone. The leader explains that some problems need to be faced, but others can be avoided. Members are asked to give examples of both types of problems. Talking about ideas for dealing with problems increases members' ability to cope more effectively.

The leader asks members to share memories about pot bellied stoves. The leader can ask where the wood or coal was put into the stove and how the ashes were taken out. Members may recall doing these chores themselves. Members from eastern cities may recall that hardened clumps of ashes called clinkers were sometimes spread on icy streets in the winter. Members may also be asked to tell how young children in the family were taught to stay away from the stove.

Sharing memories and ideas for coping builds self-esteem and feelings of belonging.

If You Can't Take the Heat, Stay Away From the Fire

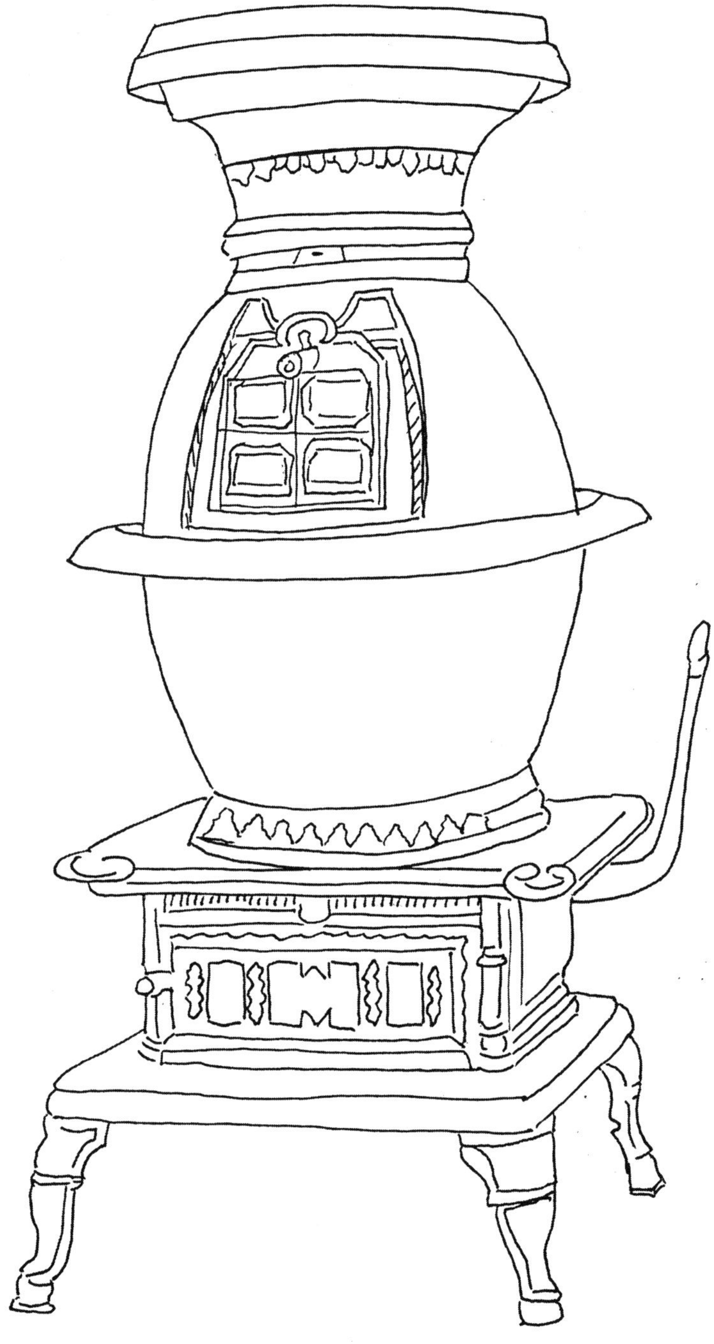

I need to stay away from: ______________________________

Exercise 26

SWEET AS PIE

Purpose:

- Share feelings about positive relationships to increase self-esteem.
- Gain insight about positive personality traits.

Materials:

One photocopy of the illustration for each group member; pencils, crayons, or fine-line colored felt pens.

Procedure:

1. While materials are distributed, members are asked to think about a person they knew that was "Sweet as Pie."
2. Members are asked to identify the picture and tell about their favorite pies.
3. The sentence fragments are read aloud and members are asked to fill in the blanks.
4. Members who like may draw or color details on the pie and plate.

Group Discussion:

Members are asked to share their pictures and memories about making and eating pie. Members share their sentence fragments about nice people they have known and characteristics that made those people nice to be around.

If dietary restrictions are an issue for some members, they may want to vent feelings about missing desserts and sweets. Sharing feelings helps to reduce frustration and depression. The leader may encourage members to share about changes that have occured over the years regarding healthy eating. For example, most members probably grew up with the idea that a breakfast of fried eggs, bacon, and toast with butter was a healthy meal.

Sweet as Pie

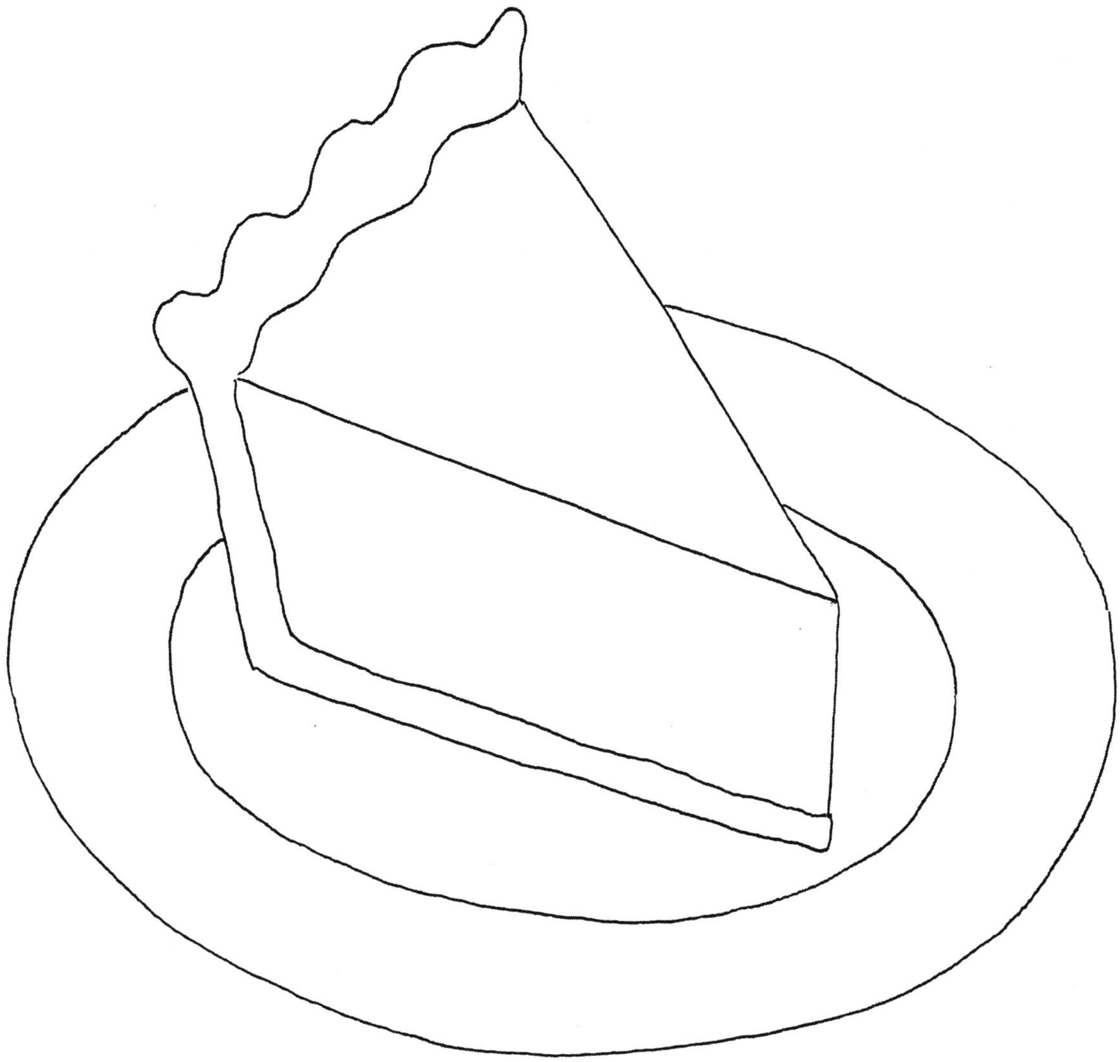

Someone I knew who was sweet as pie: ____________________

____

Something nice about that person: ____________________

____

Exercise 27

WALLFLOWER

Purpose:

- Share feelings to increase understanding of self and others.
- Share techniques to reducc isolation and withdrawal.

Materials:

One photocopy of the illustration for each group member; pencils, crayons, or fine-line colored felt pens.

Procedure:

1. Materials are passed out and members are asked to describe the term "Wallflower."
2. The sentence fragments are read aloud and members are asked to fill in the blanks.
3. Members who wish may color the picture or add wallpaper designs to the open page.

Group Discussion:

The leader explains that a wallflower is a person who is withdrawn and uninvolved in a social setting. At some time or other, most people have experienced this feeling. In some cases the person may be in a new job, new school, or new neighborhood where they are not yet acquainted. Most people have experienced feeling shy or left out at some time in their life.

Members share their pictures and sentences. The leader asks for suggestions on how to feel less lonely or left out. Suggestions might include focusing on an activity or other people to reduce self-consciousness, joining in a game or activity, or approaching one person to try to become better acquainted. Sharing common feelings increases a sense of belonging and reduces isolation.

Members share memories about wallpaper – perhaps designs they remember or when they helped hang wallpaper. Sharing background information helps to increase group cohesiveness.

Wallflower

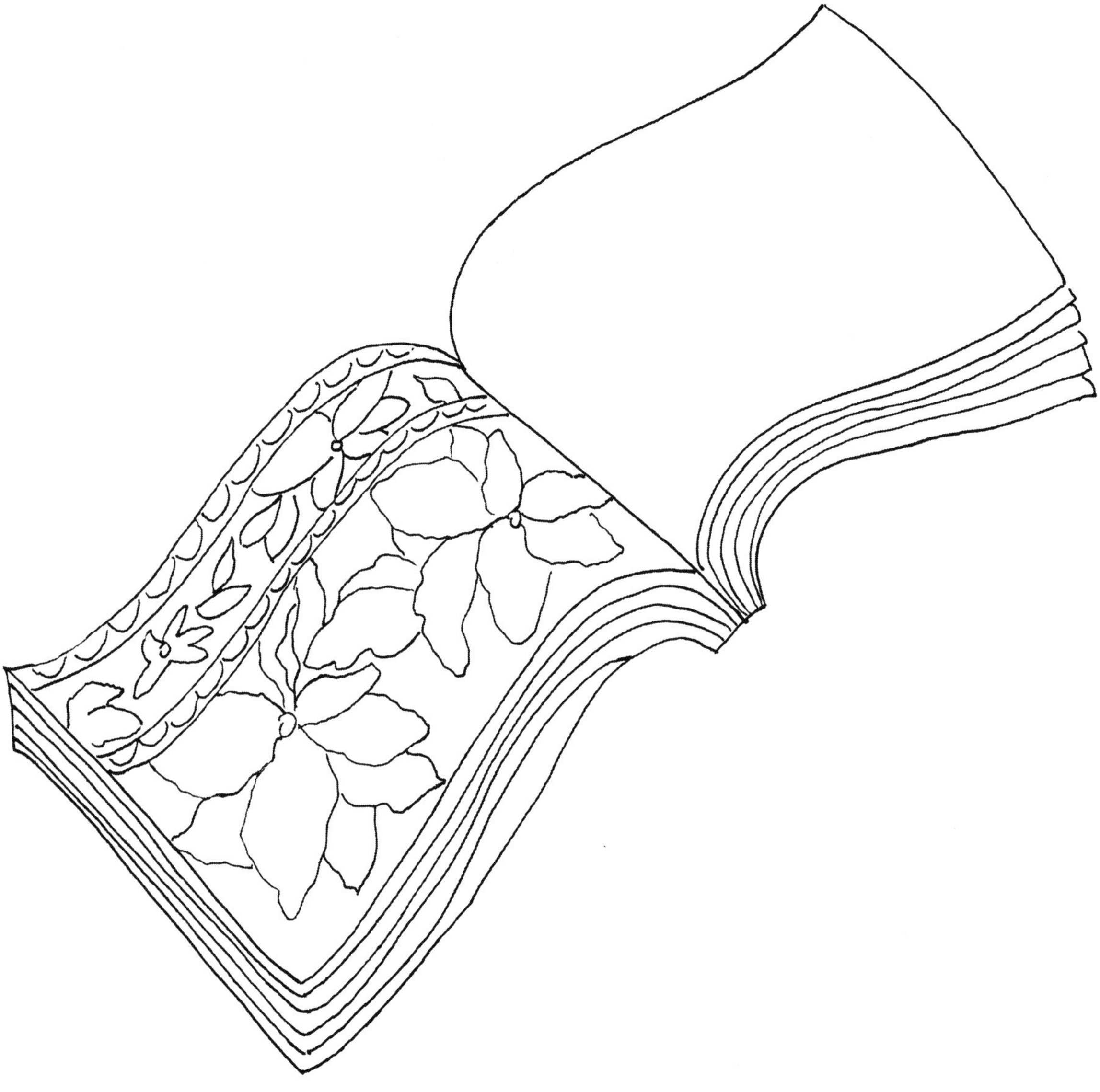

I felt like a wallflower when: ______________________________

____

I feel like participating when: ____________________________

____

Exercise 28

EXPLORING SOMETHING NEW

Purpose:

- Explore feelings about a past important news event.
- Open up possibilities for new experiences to promote flexibility in activities.

Materials:

One photocopy of the illustration for each group member; pencils, crayons, or fine-line colored felt pens.

Procedure:

1. Materials are distributed and the caption is read aloud.
2. Members are asked to recall learning that a man had landed on the moon.
3. Members are asked to fill in the blank and color the picture if they wish.

Group Discussion:

Members are asked to describe what is happening in the picture and share feelings about learning a man had landed on the moon. Members may recall how they heard the news and what was going on in their lives at the time. Sharing about a common experience helps to build group cohesiveness.

Members are asked to share their sentences about exploring something new. Some members may report trying something new in their present environment such as a new activity, meeting a new person, or trying a new hobby. The group leader encourages members to be open to new experiences. Novelty promotes cognitive growth and helps to alleviate boredom and depression.

Exploring Something New

"That's one small step for man,
one giant leap for mankind."

Neil Armstrong

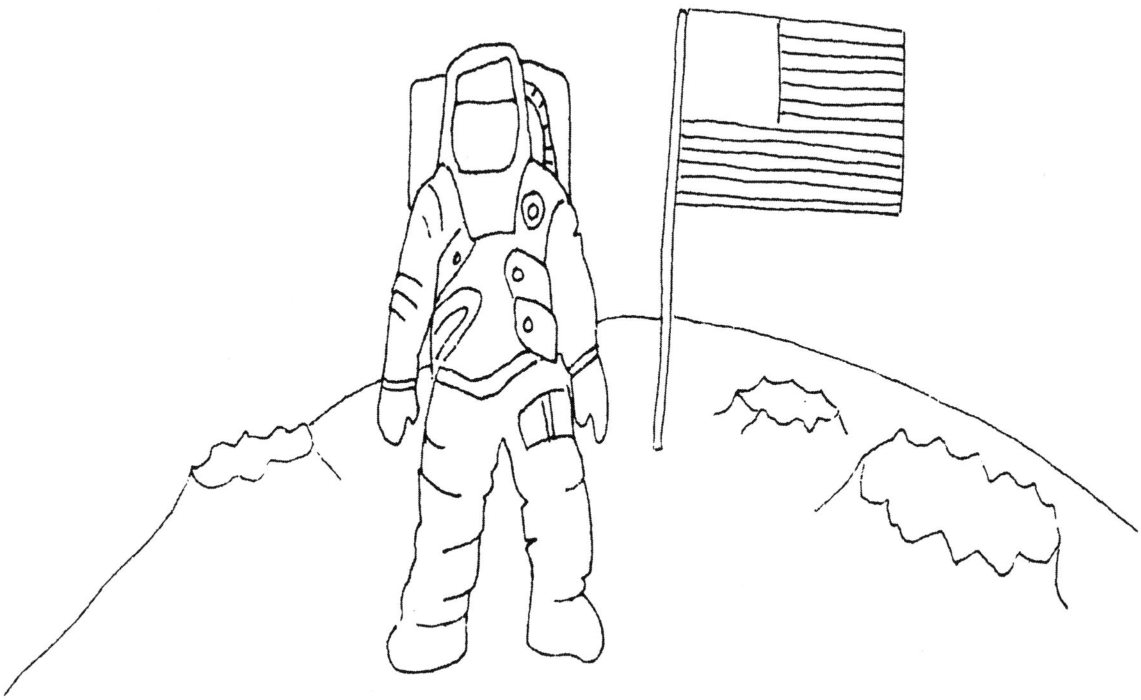

I explored something new when ____________________

____

Exercise 29

CATCH MORE FLIES WITH HONEY

Purpose:

- Share memories of past experiences to promote group cohesion.
- Gain insight about effective ways to communicate.

Materials:

One photocopy of the illustration for each group member; pencils, crayons, or fine-line colored felt pens.

Procedure:

1. Materials are distributed and the caption is read aloud.
2. Members are asked to think about the meaning of the saying, "You can catch more flies with honey than vinegar."
3. Members are asked to fill in the blank and may color the picture if they wish

Group Discussion:

Group members are asked to tell the meaning of the phrase about catching more flies with honey rather than vinegar. The leader suggests that asking for something in a nice way may get better results than being confrontational and angry. One method recommends giving a compliment first before making a request, such as complimenting the salad before asking for the meat to be more well done. Members are asked to give other ideas about asking for things in a nice way. Sharing ideas for better communication reduces frustration and increases self-esteem.

Members share their memories about bears and honey. Some members may have raised bees or retrieved honey combs themselves from wild bees. Sharing background information helps to reduce isolation.

You Can Catch More Flies With Honey Than Vinegar

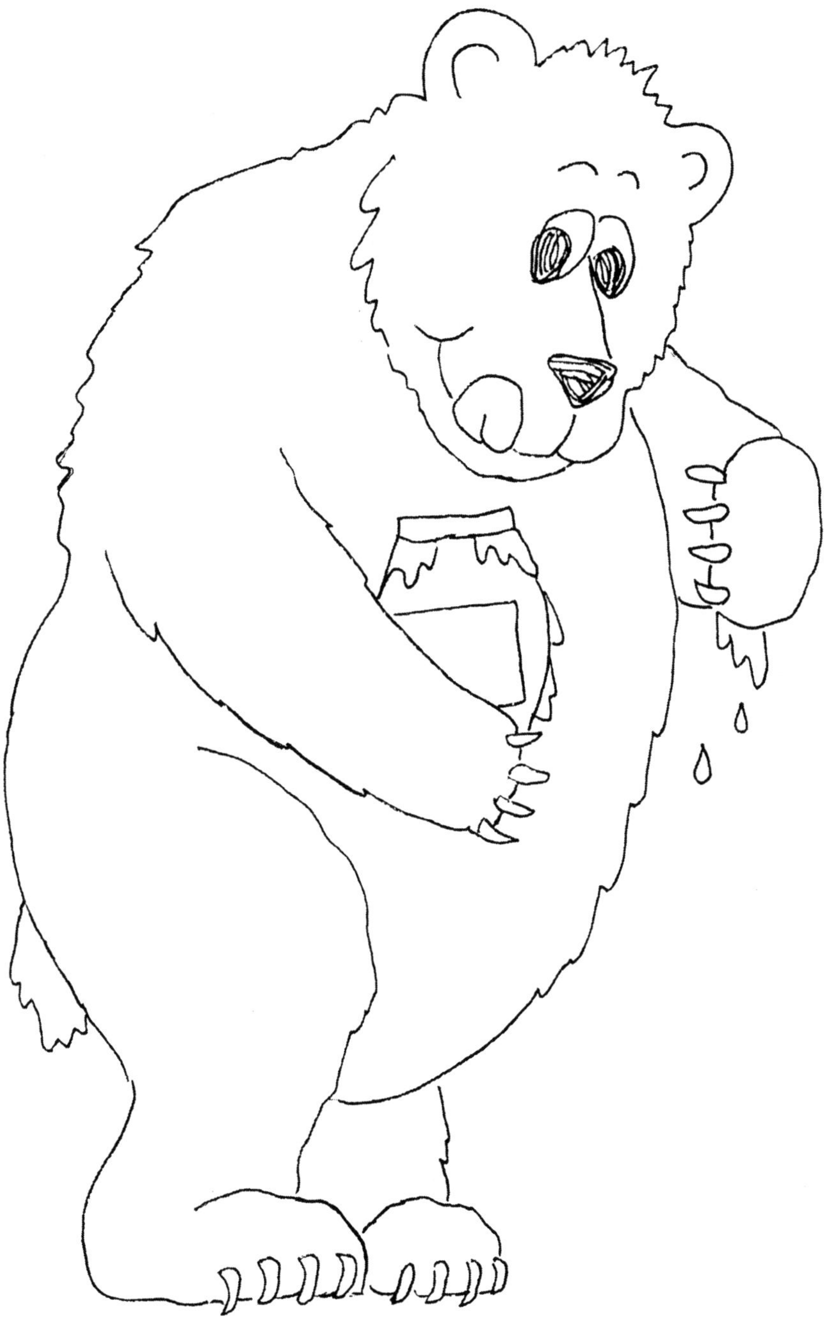

A memory I have about honey: ______________________

____

Exercise 30

SUMMERTIME

Purpose:

- Share background information about a nonthreatening topic.
- Explore positive memories to enhance identity and self-esteem.

Materials:

One photocopy of the illustration for each group member; pencils, crayons, or fine-line colored felt pens. ***Optional:*** A recording of the song "In the Good Old Summertime."

Procedure:

1. Materials are distributed and members are asked to think about summer activities.
2. Members are encouraged to color the picture and add other drawings of summer activities they enjoyed.
3. The sentence fragments are read aloud and members are asked to fill in the blanks.
4. If available, the song "In the Good Old Summertime" may be played.

Group Discussion:

Members share their pictures, memories about the song, and summer activities. Members share about summer in their home state and the meaning of summer to them at difference ages; perhaps summer meant vacations, visits with relatives, or part-time jobs. Sharing common interests and recollections increases relatedness and reduces feelings of isolation.

Members are asked to tell about their favorite season and why they like that time of year. Sharing about a nonthreatening subject builds trust and encourages participation, especially in newly formed groups.

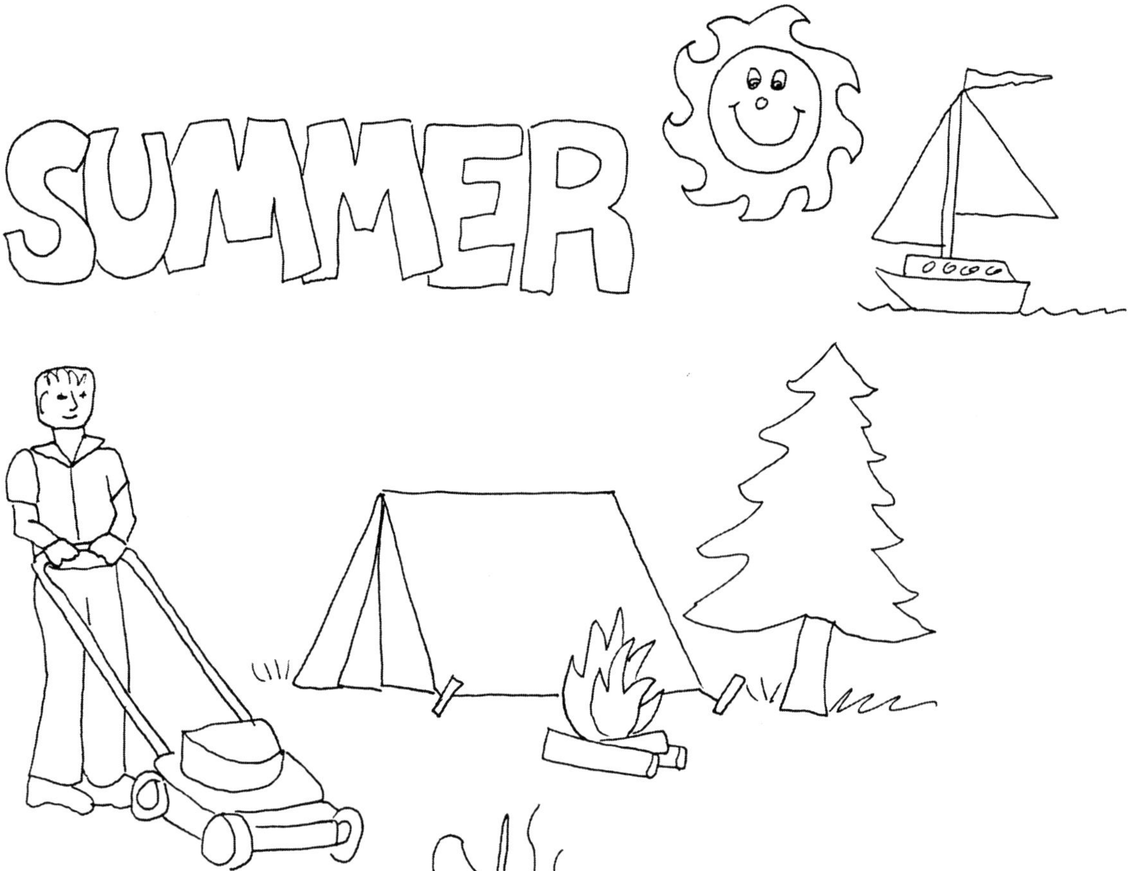

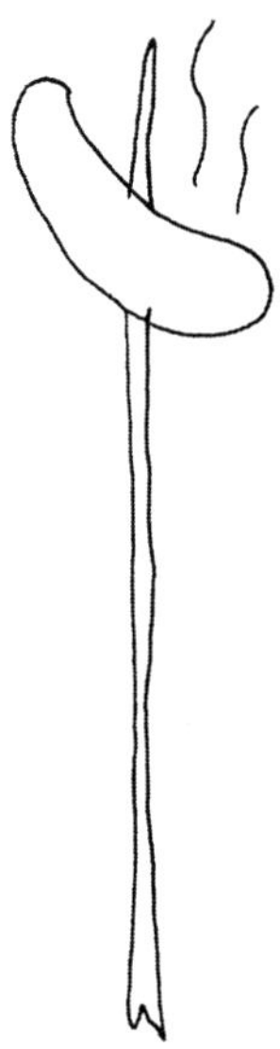

A summer activity
I enjoyed:

____

____

____

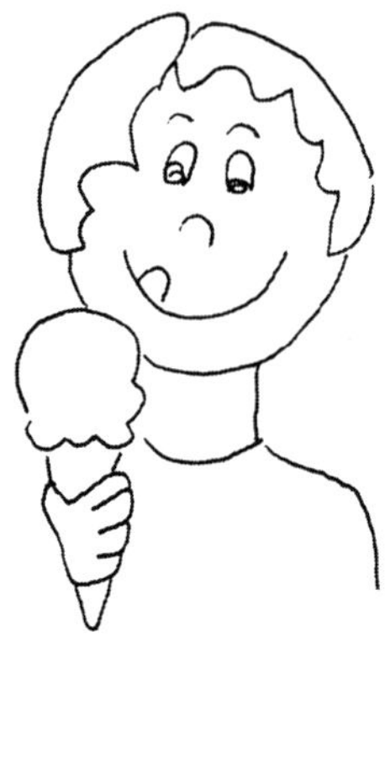

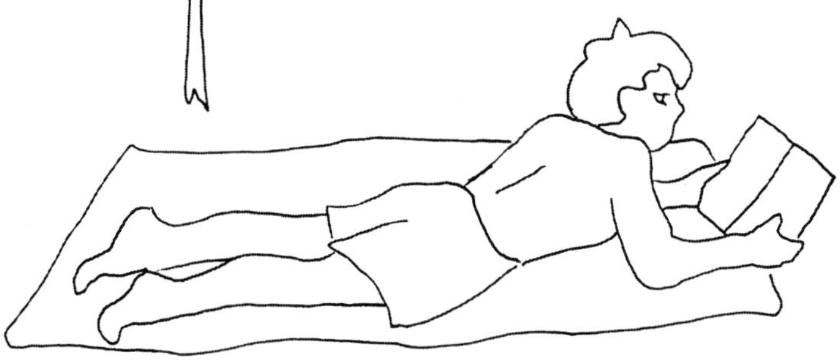

My favorite season of the year: ______________________

Exercise 31

IF WISHES WERE HORSES, BEGGARS WOULD RIDE

Purpose:

- Explore unmet needs and frustrations to increase understanding of self and others.
- Share ideas for coping with unfilled wishes in a positive way.

Materials:

One photocopy of the illustration for each group member; pencils, crayons, or fine-line colored felt pens.

Procedure:

1. While materials are distributed, members are asked to think about favorite wishes they had as children.
2. The caption is read aloud and members are asked to think about the meaning of the phrase, "If wishes were horses, beggars would ride."
3. The sentence fragments are read aloud and members are asked to fill in the blanks.
4. Members who wish may color the picture or add a rider or other details to the picture.

Group Discussion:

Members share their pictures and wishes. The leader asks if members had any envious feelings connected with the wishes and if any of the wishes came true. Sharing background information helps to build feelings of trust and belonging. Members share memories they have of horses they rode or horses they would like to have owned.

Members are asked to tell if they have heard the saying before and what it might mean. The leader explains that the caption is implying that most people have to work for what they want, not simply wish for it. The leader points out that some wishes can be translated into positive affirmations or plans of action; for example, "I wish I weighed less" could be translated into "I am enjoying healthier foods" or "I plan to eat fewer sweets." In this way wishes can sometimes stimulate a positive course of action. The leader asks members if they have personal examples of turning wishes into positive goals and how they felt about the outcome. Sharing inspirational stories inspires hope and positive coping skills.

If Wishes Were Horses, Beggars Would Ride

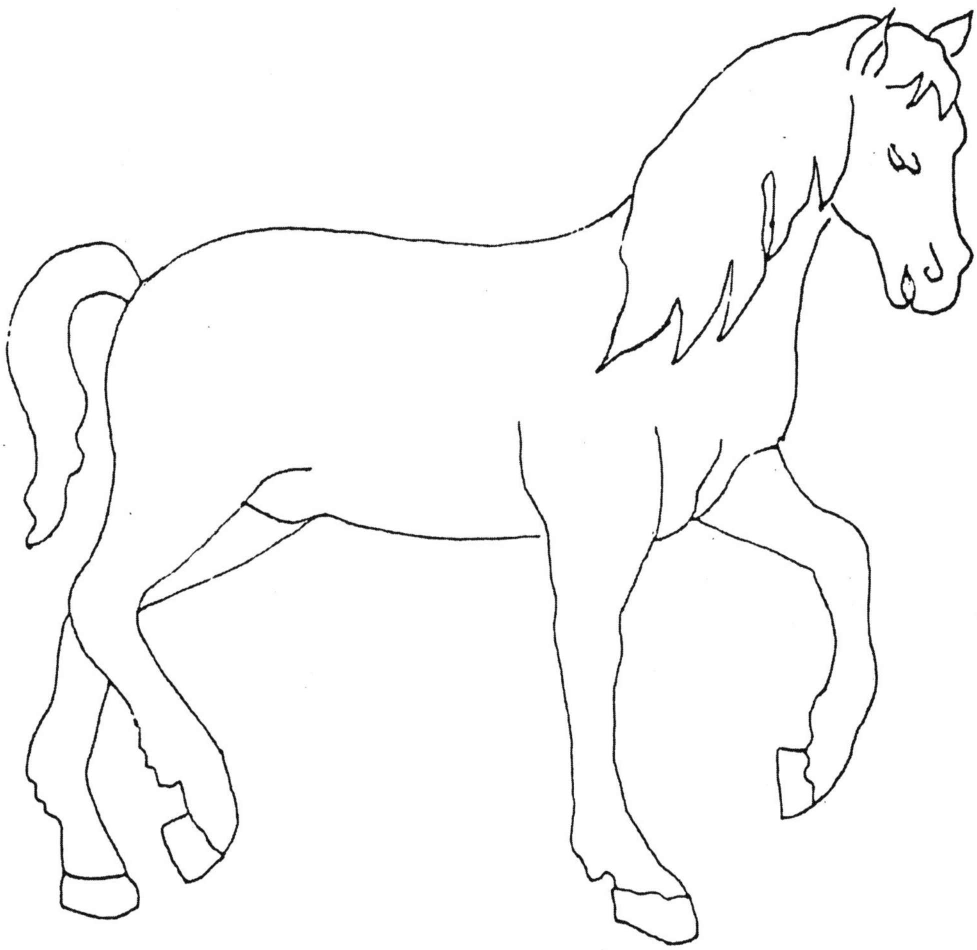

When I was a child, I wished for: ____________________

____

Sometimes I envied: __________________________________

____

Exercise 32

LET'S MAKE PEACE

Purpose:

- Raise awareness of how to coexist peacefully.
- Encourage members to act in ways that promote a peaceful environment.

Materials:

One photocopy of the illustration for each group member; pencils, crayons, or fine-line colored felt pens.

Procedure:

1. Materials are distributed and members are asked to tell what the picture represents.
2. The quotation and sentence fragment are read aloud.
3. Members who write are asked to fill in the blank.
4. Members who wish may color the picture.

Group Discussion:

The leader asks members to share recollections about Martin Luther King, Jr. and civil rights. Members may wish to share about the changes in their lives due to integration. Members are asked to share their sentences about promoting peace. The leader points out that a peaceful environment promotes health and well being. Raising awareness about the personal benefits of peace may help members to make choices which encourage peace in their living situations.

Members are asked to share memories about the Statue of Liberty and what it means to them. The leader asks if anyone has visited New York and gone up into the statue or visited other landmarks. Sharing feelings about nationalistic symbols promotes a sense of community and belonging. Sharing ideas about peace increases feelings of hope.

We have inherited a large house, a great "world house" in which we have to live together—black and white, Easterner and Westerner, Gentile and Jew, Catholic and Protestant, Moslem and Hindu—a family unduly separated in ideas, culture and interest, who, because we can never again live apart, must learn somehow to live with each other in peace.

Martin Luther King, Jr., 1967

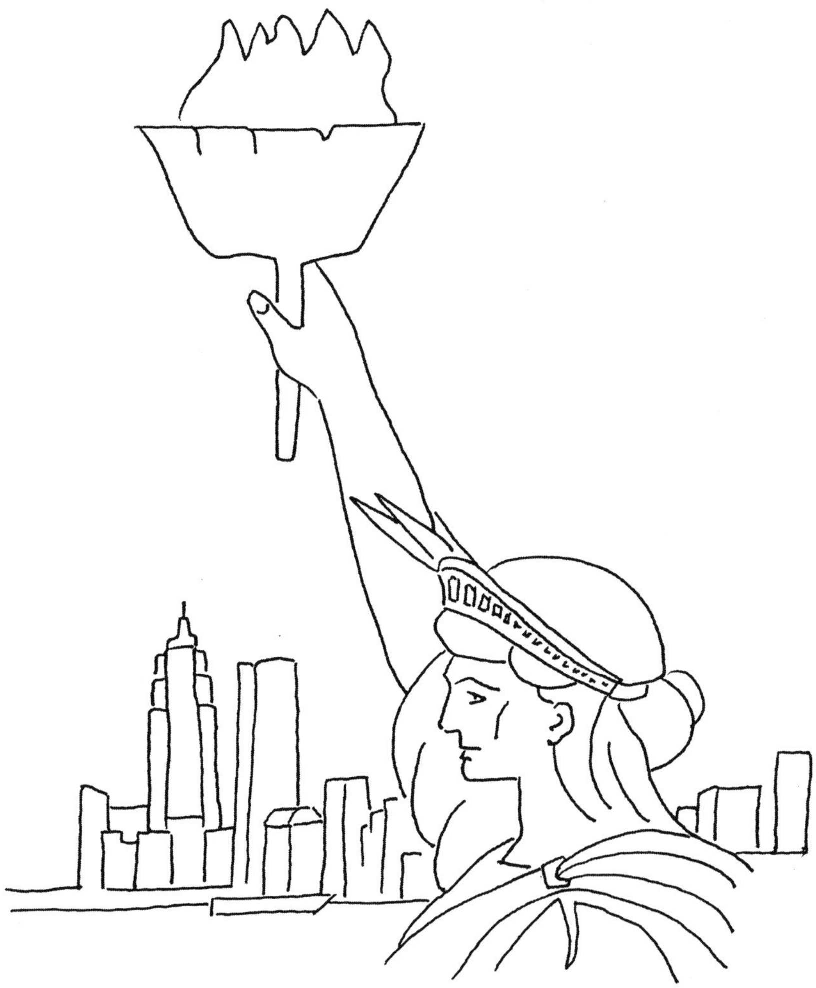

One way I could help to make my living situation more peaceful: ______________________________

____

Exercise 33

PLEASE MR. POSTMAN

Purpose:

- Share memories about important communications.
- Encourage communication to reduce feelings of isolation.

Materials:

One photocopy of the illustration for each group member; pencils, crayons, or fine-line colored felt pens. ***Optional:*** A recording of the song, "Please Mr. Postman."

Procedure:

1. Materials are distributed and the caption is read aloud.
2. Members are asked to identify the pictures and think of memories about written communication.
3. The sentence fragments are read aloud and members are asked to fill in the blanks. Those who wish may add pictures associated with writing or color the picture.
4. The song, "Please Mr. Postman" may be played if available.

Group Discussion:

Members share their memories about the illustration of the manual typewriter and the early computer. Members may tell how they learned to type and share memories about the manual typewriter, such as dealing with keys sticking, mistakes, and changing the ribbon. Members who use computers may share their experience of writing on the computer or their frustrations using computers. Some members may share about their experiences with early computers, e-mail, or Facebook.

Members are asked if they recall the song, "Please Mr. Postman" about someone waiting for a letter. Members share their pictures and tell about letters they received and people they would write to. The leader reflects on the fact that people communicate less and less by letter as opposed to phone, text, and e-mail. Group members share feelings about these current trends. Some members may share stories about reconnecting with someone from the past. The leader encourages members to reach out to someone with whom they would like to connect. Ideas might include calling distant friends or family members or sending a thank-you card to someone who has been helpful. At a future group meeting, members share about their experiences of trying to contact someone and any replies they received. Encouraging communication reduces isolation and self-absorption.

Please Mr. Postman

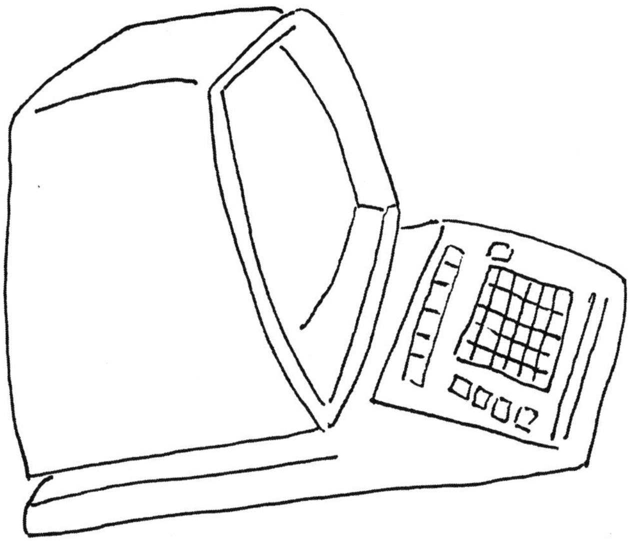

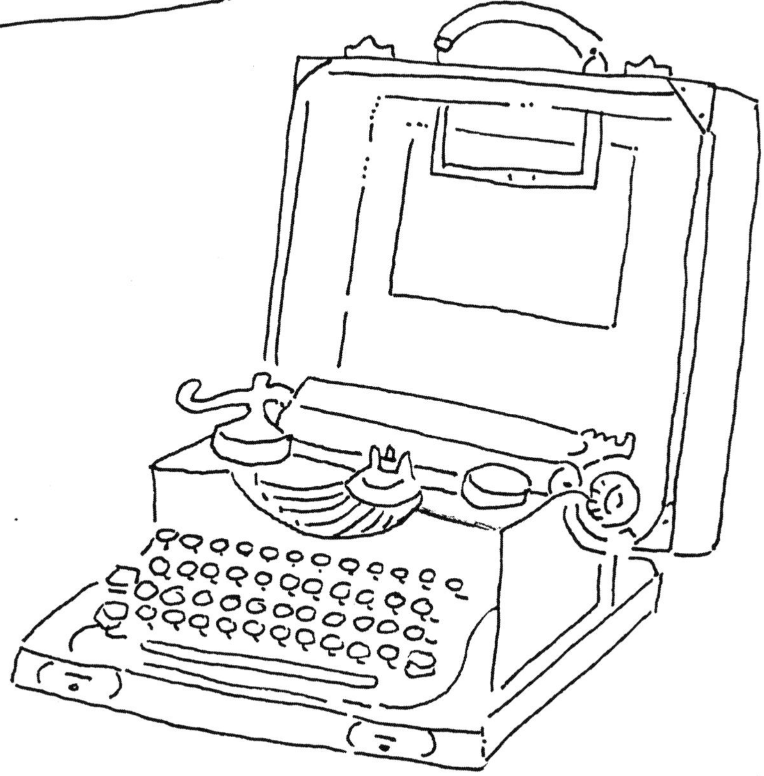

An important letter I received: ______________________

____

If I wrote to someone, I would write to: ______________

____

Exercise 34

WEARING DIFFERENT HATS

Purpose:

- Share personal history to strengthen identity and self-esteem.
- Practice listening to others to promote understanding and relatedness.

Materials:

One photocopy of the illustration for each group member; pencils, crayons, or fine-line colored felt pens.

Procedure:

1. Materials are passed out and the caption is read aloud.
2. Members are asked to tell what they think the saying, "Wearing different hats" could mean.
3. Members are asked to circle, color, or draw different hats they have worn.
4. The sentence fragment is read aloud and members who write are asked to fill in the blank with a hat they have worn or a different role they have played in life.

Group Discussion:

Members are asked to share their pictures and memories about the hats pictured in the illustration or one they have drawn. Group members may recall when hats were an important part of a person's wardrobe. The leader can ask members if they had a favorite hat, what color the hat was, and whether it had feathers or other special decorations.

The leader explains that wearing different hats can mean functioning in different roles. For example, a person might work as a teacher and also function as a wife and mother. Members are asked to share about different roles they have played in life.

Members are encouraged to ask each other questions about the information that has been shared to practice showing interest in other peoples' lives. Sharing information and listening to others increases feelings of belonging.

Wearing Different Hats

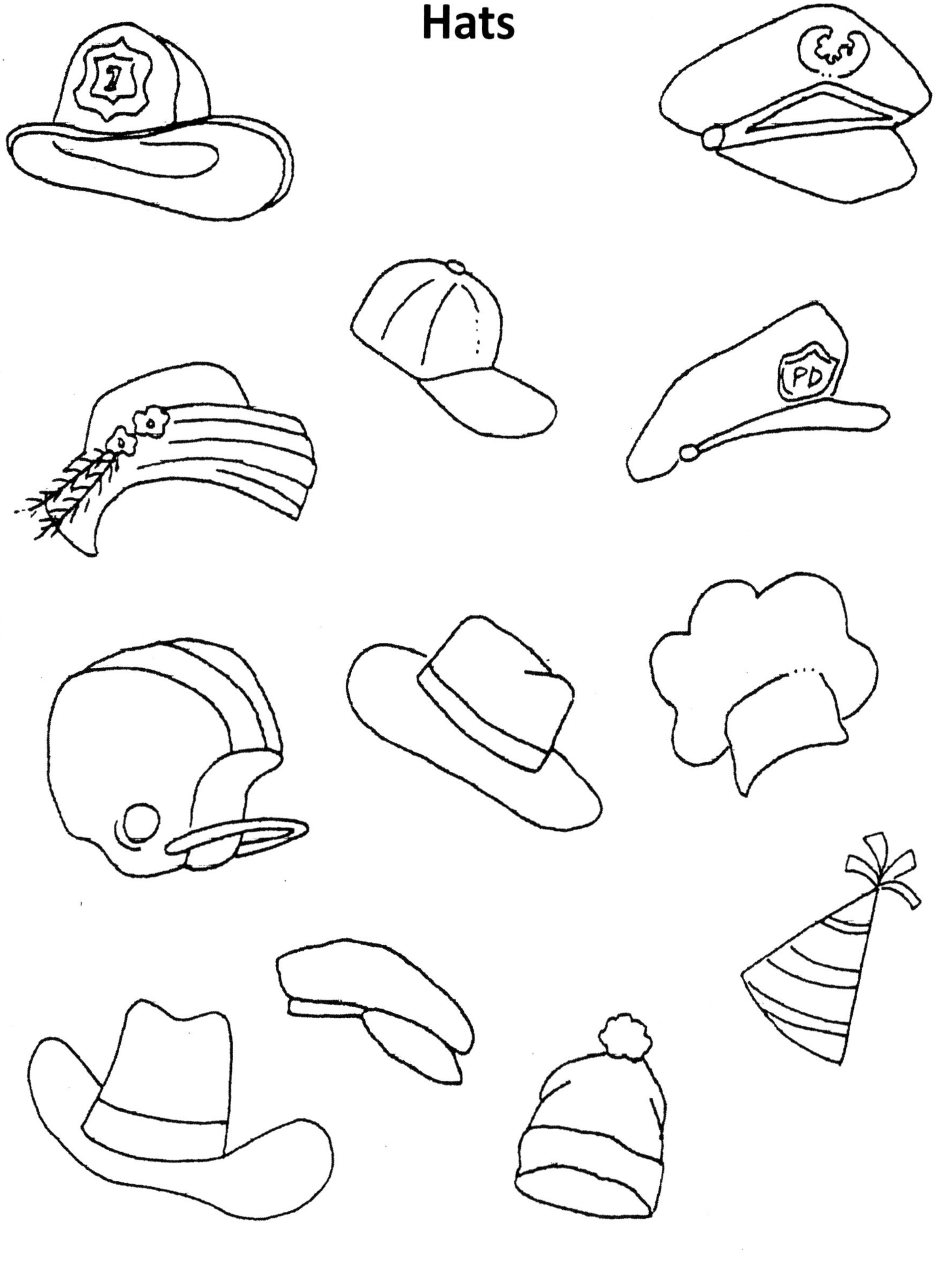

A different hat I've worn: ______________________________

Exercise 35

BUMPY ROADS

Purpose:

- Open up feelings about difficult times.
- Share ideas about how to cope with hard times.

Materials:

One photocopy of the illustration for each group member; pencils, crayons, or fine-line colored felt pens.

Procedure:

1. Materials are distributed and the caption and sentence fragments are read aloud.
2. Members are asked to tell what the saying "Life was a bumpy road" means.
3. Members are asked to give examples of times when life seemed like a bumpy road.
4. Members who write are asked to fill in the blanks with difficult times and advice on coping.
5. Members who wish may color the picture and draw someone behind the wheel of the car.

Group Discussion:

Members share their illustrations and sentences. Sharing feelings about difficult times helps to increase group cohesion. Listening to advice from others on how to cope with hard times may increase members' ideas for handling their own difficulties.

To stimulate reminiscence, the leader asks if members can identify the car in the illustration. The leader explains that the picture resembles a 1932 Plymouth, known as a Sport Roadster. Members are told that the Chrysler vehicles in the early 1930's were mass produced and used four-wheel hydraulic brakes and special shock absorbers to provide a more comfortable ride. Members are asked if they recall early bumpy roads or cobblestone streets. Sharing memories builds feelings of belonging and increases a sense of identity.

Bumpy Roads

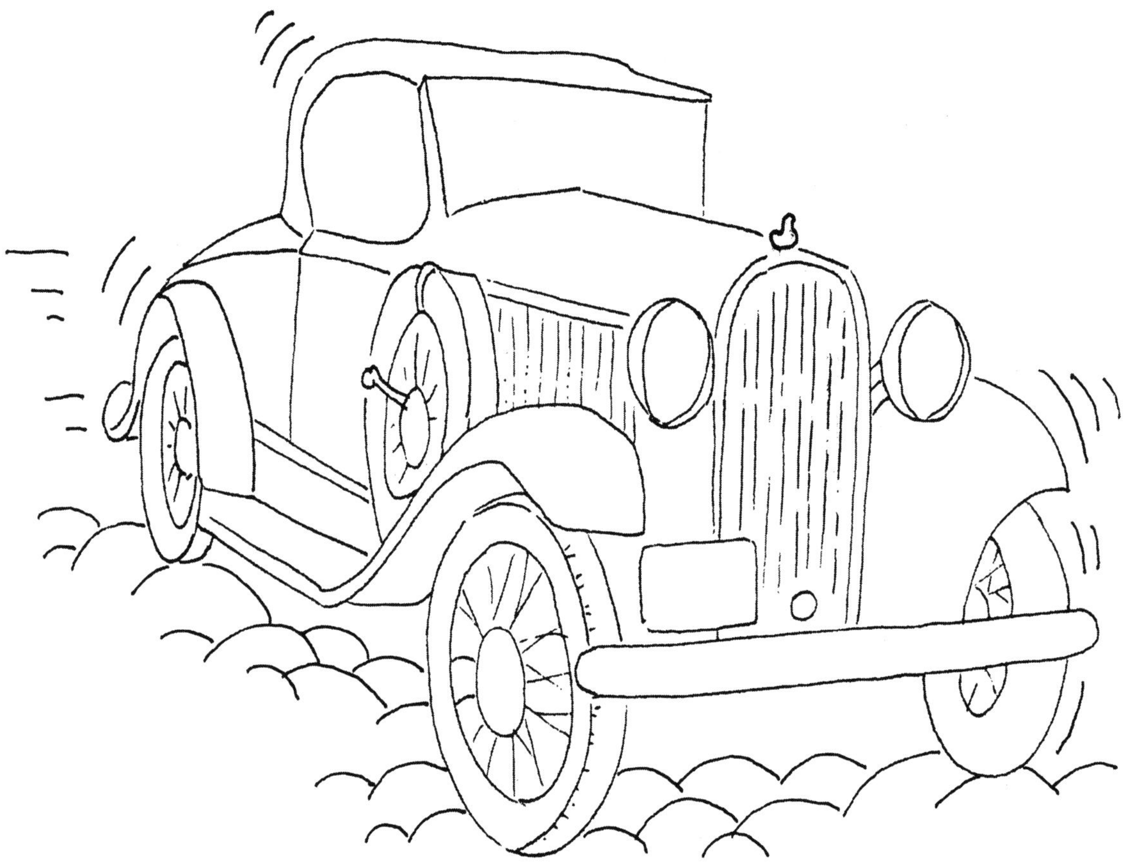

Life was a bumpy road for me when: ____________________

____

____

My best advice for making it through hard times is to: _____

____

____

Exercise 36

MOODS AND THE WEATHER

Purpose:

- Open up feelings about how weather affects group members' moods.
- Increase undcrstanding of how different ways of thinking affect a person's mood.

Materials:

One photocopy of the illustration for each group member; pencils, crayons, or fine-line colored felt pens. ***Optional:*** A recording of the song "Singing in the Rain."

Procedure:

1. Materials are distributed and members are asked to tell what famous song the illustration might represent.
2. The sentence fragments are read aloud and members who write are asked to fill in the blanks with their ideas about rainy weather.
3. Members who wish may color the picture.
4. If available, a recording of the song "Singing in the Rain" may be played.

Group Discussion:

The leader asks group members who the singer in the illustration could be and what song and movie the picture might depict. If group members are not able to guess the answers, the leader explains that the illustration resembles Gene Kelly in "Singing in the Rain," a song and movie featuring the famous dancer and singer of the 1930's. The leader explains that the song tells about a man being so happy that he is singing in the rain with no regard for the weather. Members are asked to share memories about the song or movie.

Group members show their pictures and read their sentences. The leader points out that finding something pleasant to do may improve a person's mood even on a gloomy, rainy day. Sharing memories and ideas for coping reduces isolation and increases group cohesion.

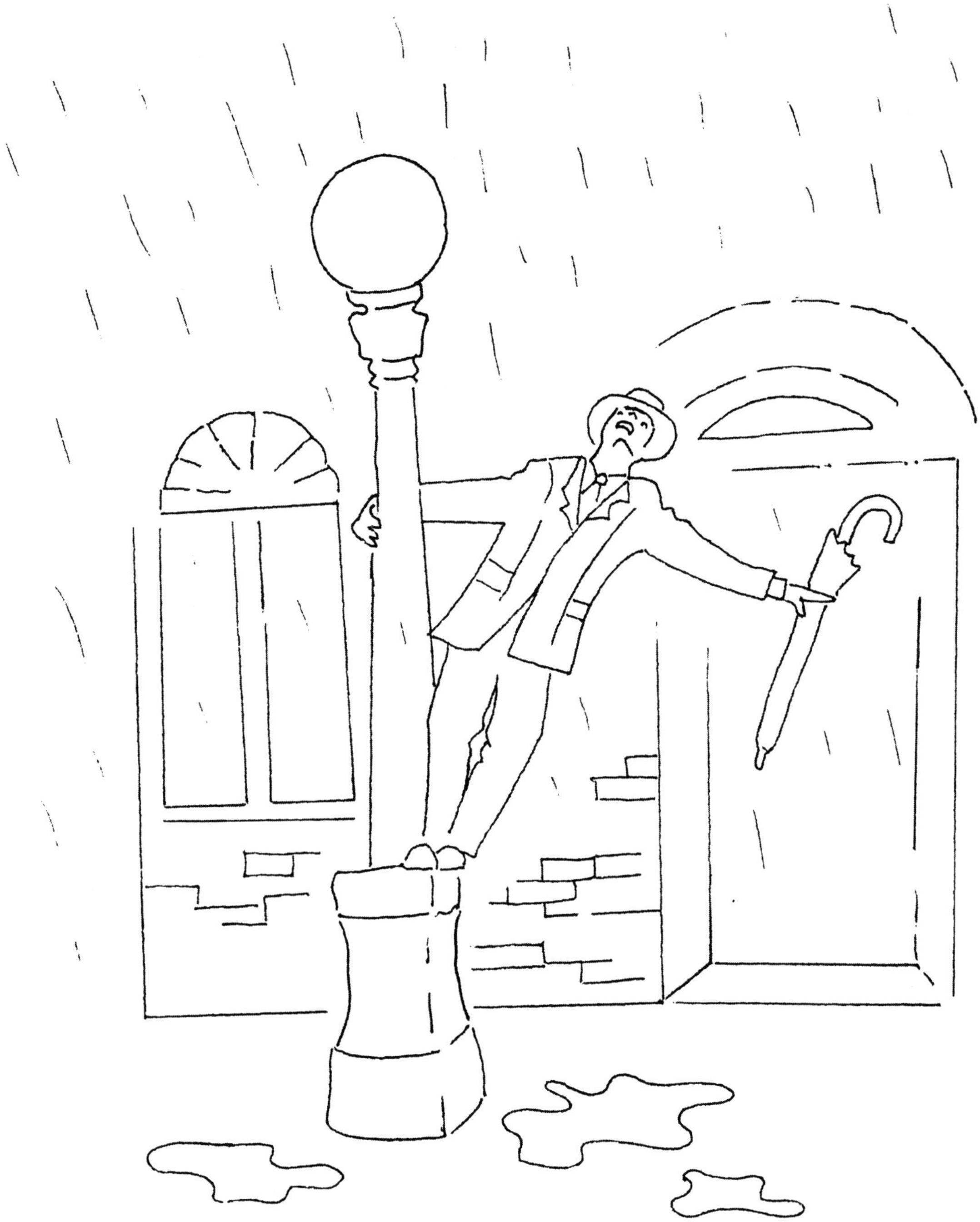

The effect rainy weather has on my mood: ____________

____

What I like to do on a rainy day: ________________

____

Exercise 37

TAKE ME OUT TO THE BALLGAME

Purpose:

- Share accomplishments and interests to enhance identity and self-esteem.
- Review positive coping skills to reduce stress and frustration.

Materials:

One copy of the illustration for each member; pencils and colored felt pens. ***Optional:*** A recording of the song "Take Me Out to the Ballgame."

Procedure:

1. Materials are distributed and members are asked to think about sports they have played or watched.
2. Sentence fragments are read aloud and members who write are asked to fill in the blanks.
3. Members who wish may color the picture and add drawings of sports equipment.
4. If available, a recording of the song "Take Me Out to the Ball game" is played.

Group Discussion:

Members are asked to share memories about the song or going to ballgames. Members share their pictures and sentences about sports they enjoyed watching or playing. Sharing interests and background information increases self-esteem and promotes interest in others.

The leader asks members to share things they learned from playing sports. Ideas might include working as a team, learning to be a good sport, accepting one's limits, and having respect for authority. The leader asks if anyone can give a recent example of using some of these coping skills in their daily life. Sharing coping skills reduces frustration and isolation.

Members are asked for current ideas for watching or playing games. Raising awareness of opportunities for enjoyable activity promotes motivation and interest in living.

Take Me Out
To the Ball Game

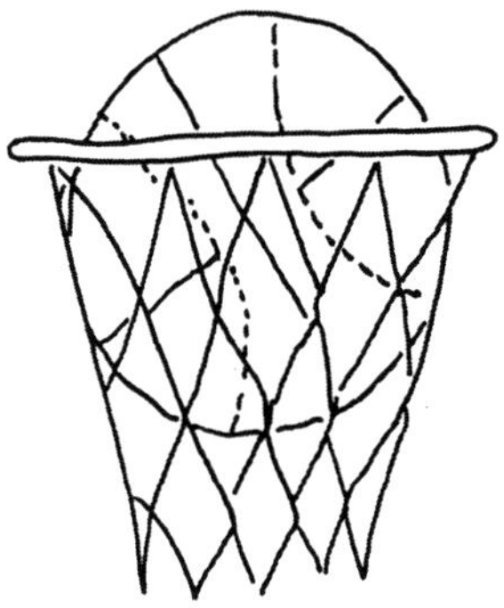

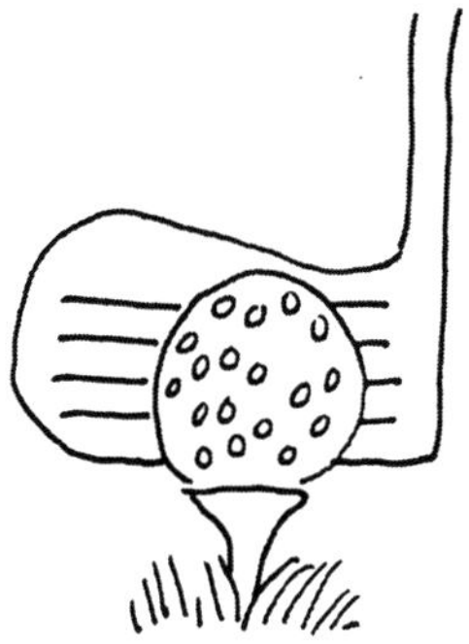

A sport I liked
playing or watching:

____

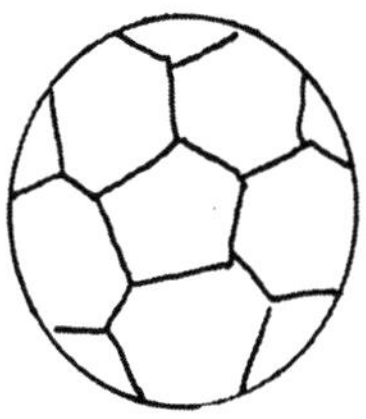

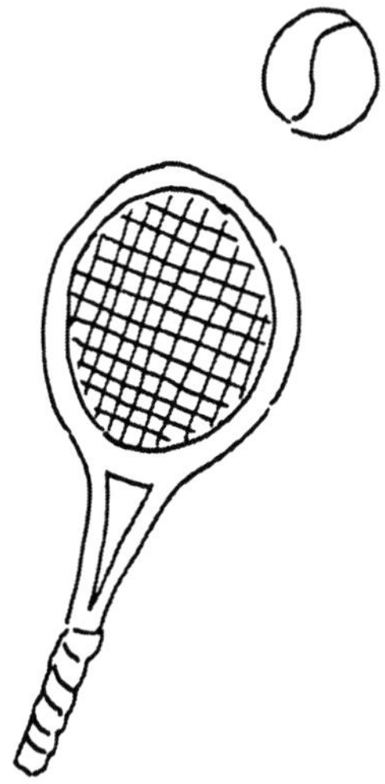

Some things I learned
from playing sports:

____

____

____

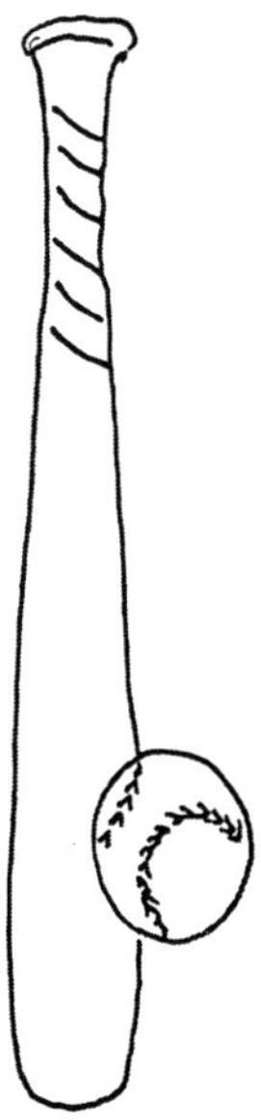

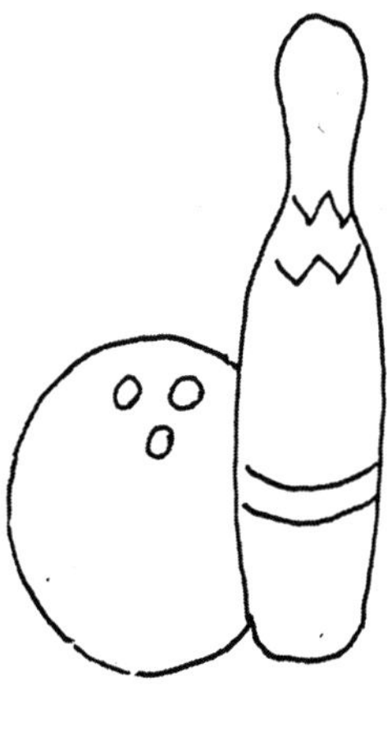

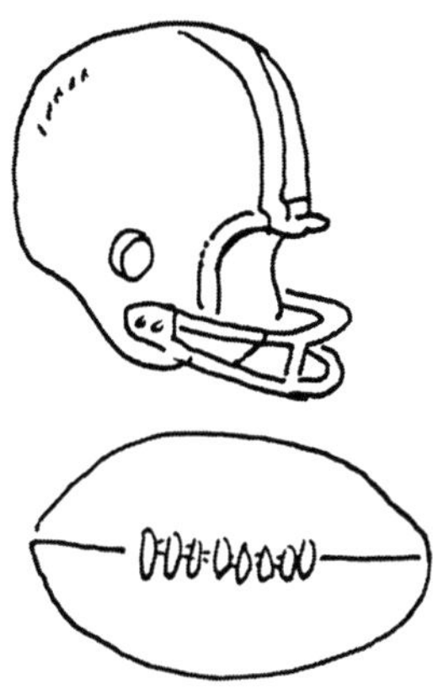

Exercise 38

FOODS AND FEELINGS

Purpose:

- Stimulate positive reminiscence about foods.
- Explore feelings about current menus and diets.

Materials:

One photocopy of the illustration for each group member; pencils, crayons, or fine-line colored felt pens.

Procedure:

1. While handing out materials, the leader asks members to think about home cooked meals they have enjoyed.
2. Those who wish may draw favorite home cooked foods, and color the picture.
3. The words are read aloud and members are asked to complete the sentence.

Group Discussion:

Members are asked to share memories about the illustration of a woman making cupcakes or muffins. The leader asks members to share their sentences, pictures, and memories about baking and cooking. They may share about how they learned to cook and who did the cooking in their family.

Members are encouraged to share feelings about their current diet, both positive and negative. Ideas for coping with dietary issues might include communicating likes and dislikes to dietary personnel and learning more about the purpose of dietary choices and restrictions. Sharing feelings and ideas for coping reduces isolation and frustration.

Sharing ideas about a familiar subject in a nonthreatening format helps group members to express feelings, develop trust, and build feelings of community.

Foods and Feelings

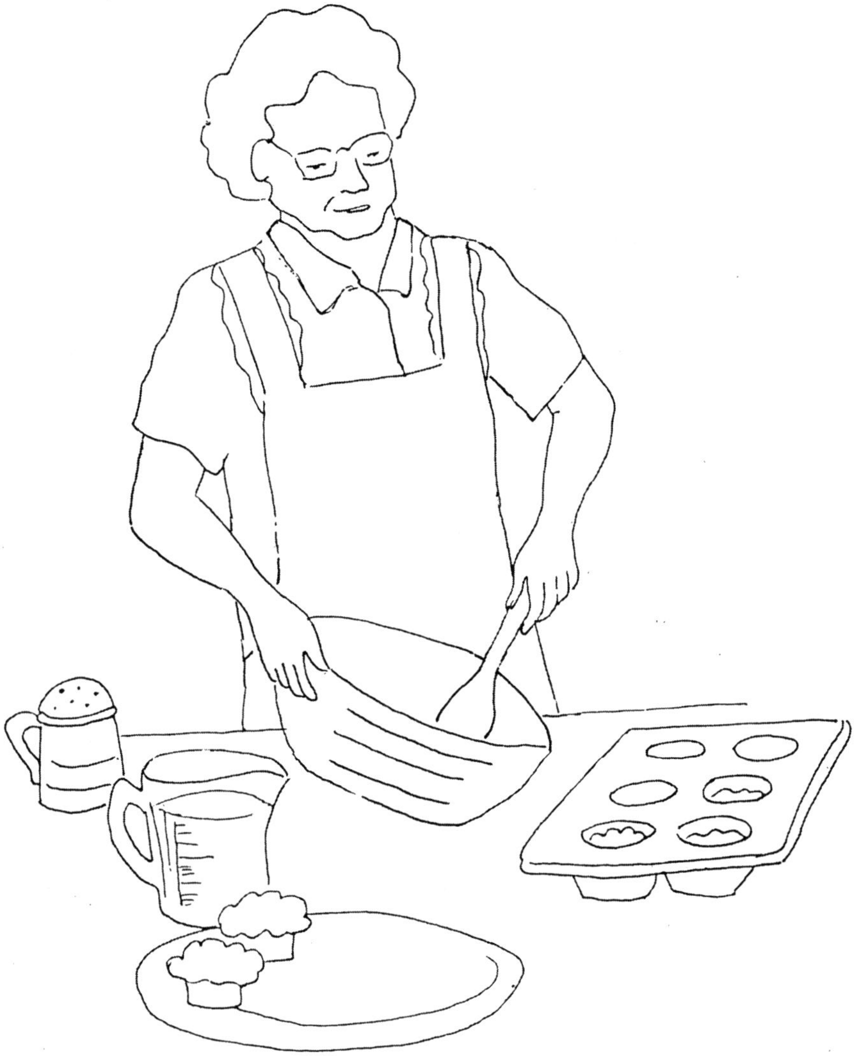

A home-cooked meal I like: ______________________________

____

Food I like now: ____

If I could change the food I eat now I would: _____________

____

____

Exercise 39

COMMUNICATION

Purpose:

- Express feelings regarding communication in the past and present.
- Provide group support for feelings of loneliness and isolation.

Materials:

One photocopy of the illustration for each group member; pencils, crayons, or fine-line colored felt pens.

Procedure:

1. Materials are distributed and the leader asks group members to share memories about the phones in the illustration. Members may recall using rotary dial phones before cell phones were available.
2. Members are encouraged to complete the sentences. Some members may wish to color the illustration or draw the face of a person they would like to talk to next to the receiver.

Group Discussion:

Members share their illustrations and ideas about people they would like to contact. Members are asked to tell about losing contact with people in their lives and how they feel about these experiences. The leader asks the group for ideas on ways to maintain contact with others.

This exercise is helpful in stimulating interest in communication and allowing ventilation of feelings regarding loss and isolation.

Variations:

Group members are encouraged to plan one way to communicate with someone they would like to contact. In later meetings, members may wish to share their experiences.

Communication

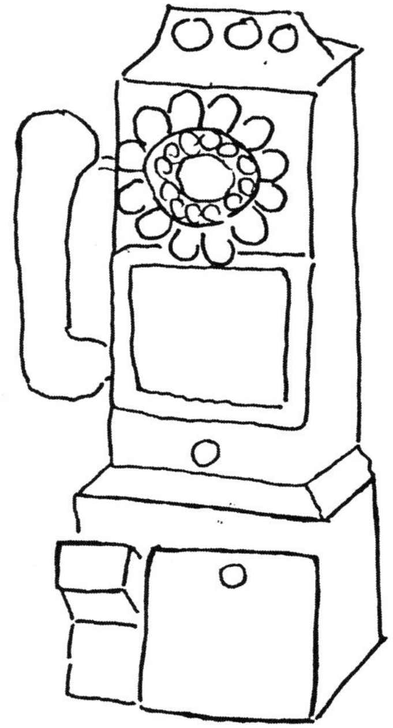

I would like to talk to: ______________________________

I would talk about: ________________________________

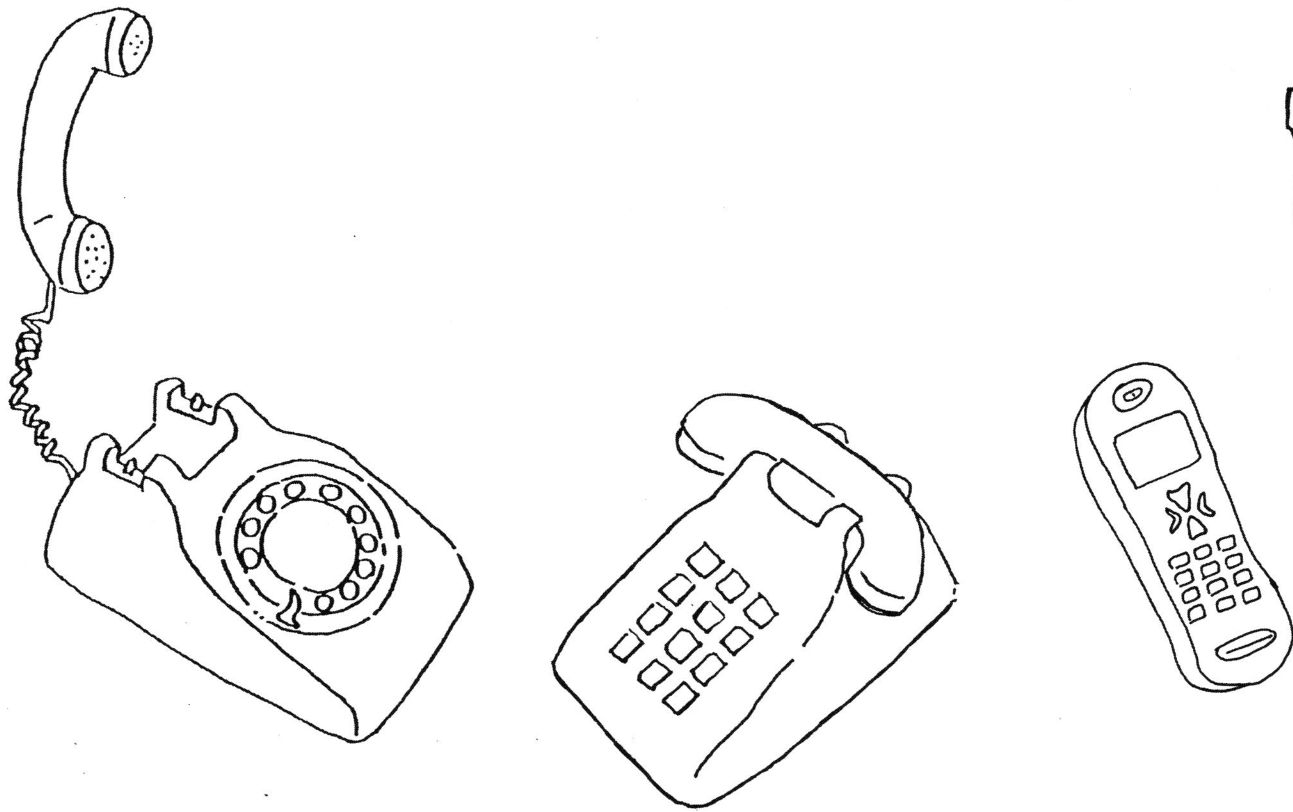

Exercise 40

ROMANTIC MOMENTS

Purpose:

- Share personal memories and feelings to increase a sense of belonging.
- Practice reminiscence in a group setting to strengthen identity and self-esteem.

Materials:

One photocopy of the illustration for each group member; crayons and pencils.

Procedure:

1. While materials are distributed, members are asked to think about romantic moments in their lives.
2. The sentences are read aloud and members are asked to fill in the blanks. Members are told they can write about events in their own lives or romantic scenes from a book or movie.
3. Members who wish may draw favorite candies in the box and color the box.

Group Discussion:

Members share their illustrations and sentences. If members share frustrations or feelings of loss about a disappointing romance, the leader and other group members offer support by expressing feelings of understanding and empathy.

This exercise increases group cohesiveness by stimulating reminiscence and promoting expression of feelings. Participants may discover that other group members share their interest in particular movie stars. Sharing common interests helps to build relatedness.

Romantic Moments

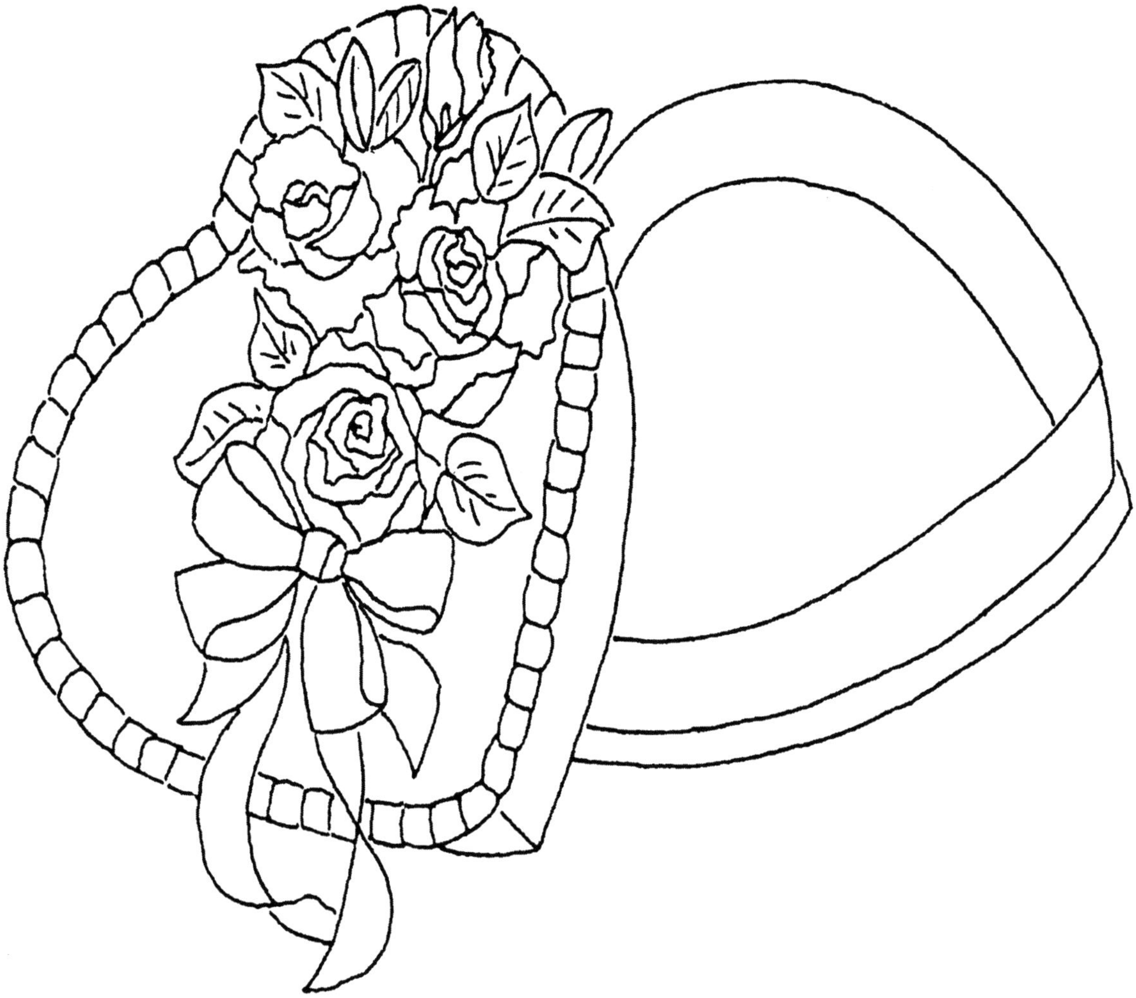

____________________________ was a very romantic person.

A favorite romantic memory of mine: ____________________

____

____

____

____

A romantic movie star: _________________________________

Exercise 41

TRANSPORTATION

Purpose:

- Encourage expression of feelings about mobility and independence.
- Promote active listening and awareness of the feelings of others.
- Practice giving and receiving group support for feelings of frustration.

Materials:

One photocopy of the illustration for each member; pencils, crayons, or fine-line colored felt pens.

Procedure:

1. Members are asked to think about their favorite car while materials are distributed.
2. The sentence fragments are read aloud and members are asked to fill in the blanks.
3. Members who wish may draw someone in the cars, color the cars, or draw a favorite car design of their own.

Group Discussion:

Members share their illustrations and sentences. Members who did not drive are asked how they managed transportation. Members are asked to share memories about the Packard and Volkswagon Beetle in the picture. They may have other stories about how they learned to drive and about cars they drove or wanted to drive.

Members are asked how transportation is managed where they live. If feelings of frustration about transportation are expressed, the leader and group members may provide group support by validating feelings and offering suggestions for coping.

This exercise is beneficial in stimulating group support and encouraging ventilation of frustrations about declines in independence.

Transportation

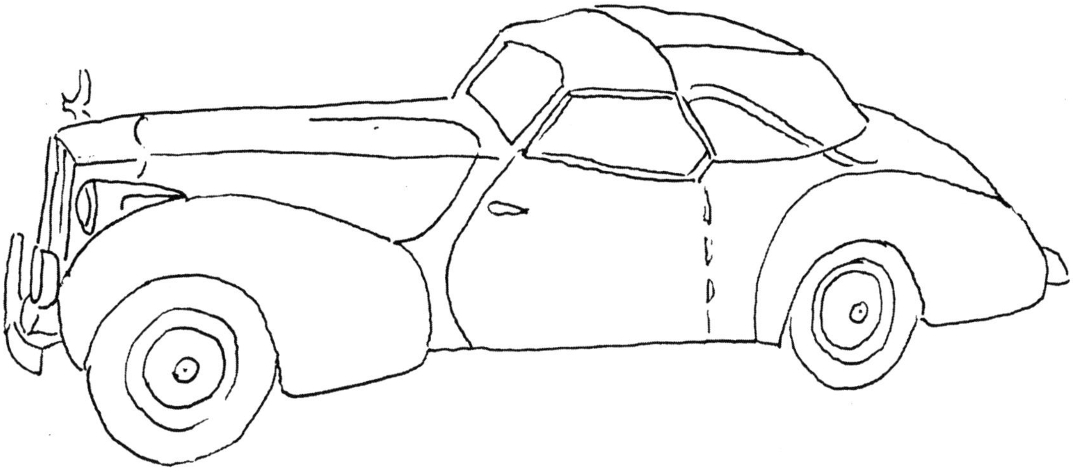

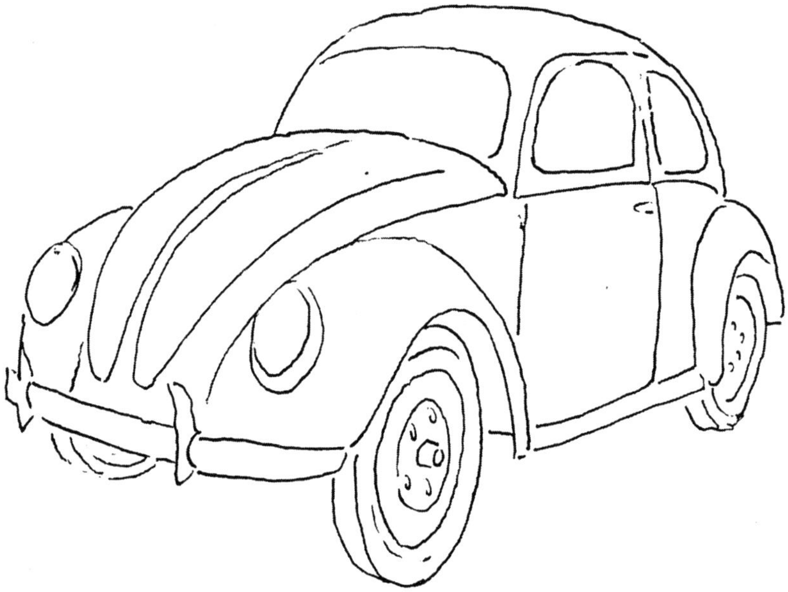

My favorite car: ______________________________________

____

A car I would like to have driven: ______________________

____

Exercise 42

GROUP POEM

Objectives:

- Promote expression of feelings and enhance creativity.
- Raise self-esteem and group morale by contributing to a collective creative project.

Materials:

One photocopy of Group Poem worksheet for each member; pencils. ***Optional:*** posterboard, scissors, glue, and old magazines.

Procedure:

1. The leader points out that we are each unique in the way we experience and express feelings.
2. Materials are distributed and the leader explains that the photocopy will be used to create a group poem.
3. Members are instructed to finish the sentences on the worksheet. The leader may help those who have difficulty writing.

Group Discussion:

Members take turns reading and discussing their contributions. Permission is asked of the members to combine their expressions into a poem. Using the Group Leader's Worksheet, the leader arranges the various ideas supplied by the members to complete a poem. Copies are distributed to the members acknowledging their special contributions.

This exercise increases feelings of belonging and promotes good self-esteem. Members are often pleased by how their contributions add to the effectiveness of the poem.

Variation:

The group poem can be displayed on posterboard. Pictures from old magazines can be cut out and glued around a copy of the poem to illustrate the ideas in the poem.

Group Poem

Fall leaves remind me of:

____

When winter comes, I feel:

____

When spring comes, I hope for:

____

My favorite flower:

____

It's good to think about:

____

Group Leader's Worksheet for Group Poem

Fall leaves remind me of:

When winter comes, I feel:

When spring comes, I hope for:

My favorite flower:

It's good to think about:

Exercise 43

COPING WITH PAIN

Purpose:

- Promote healthy mechanisms for coping with pain or disability.
- Increase understanding of and group support for meeting health challenges.

Materials:

One photocopy of the illustration for each group member; crayons.

Procedure:

1. Materials are distributed and the leader explains that the figures in the illustration represent the front and back of a patient arriving and leaving a doctor's appointment.
2. Members are asked to think about physical pain they have experienced. Members are instructed to select colors to represent pain or limitation they experience or have experienced and color the corresponding part on the figures in the drawing.

Group Discussion:

Members present their figures and tell about the pain in the areas they have colored. Members are asked what they do to cope with pain or disability. Their answers may give other group members ideas on how to cope.

This exercise promotes empathy and bonding in older populations who are particularly stressed by physical problems. Participants may become more aware of the physical challenges others face and consequently develop greater empathy for others.

Coping With Pain

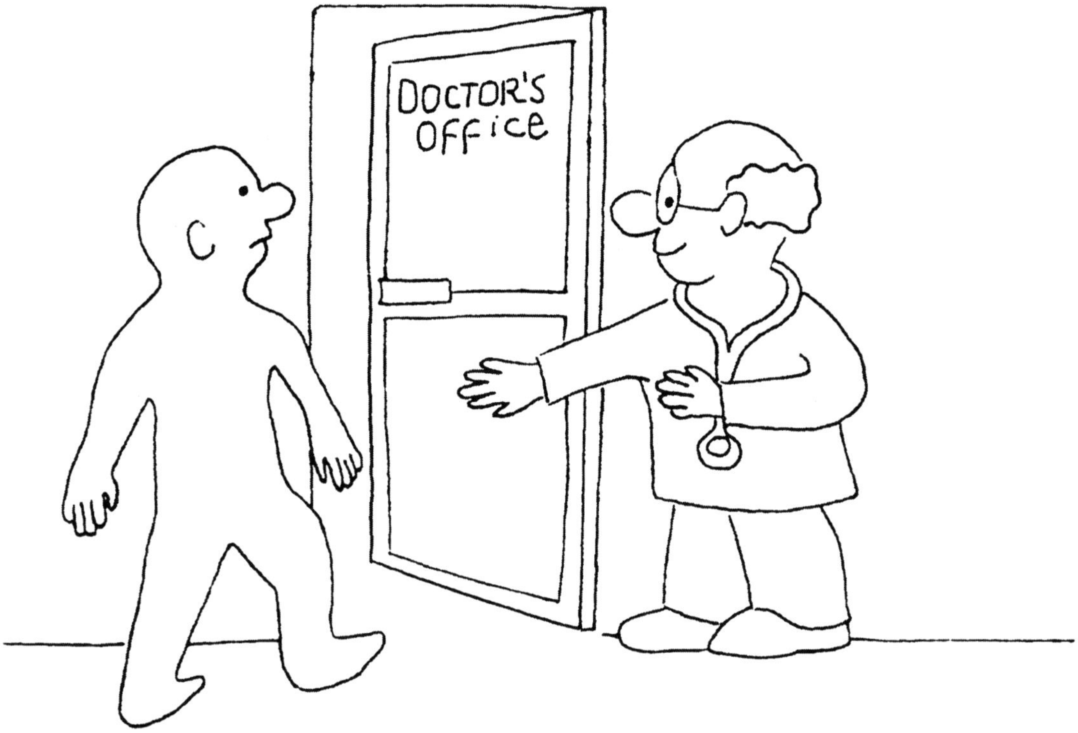

Physical pain that bothers me the most: ______________________________

____

____

____

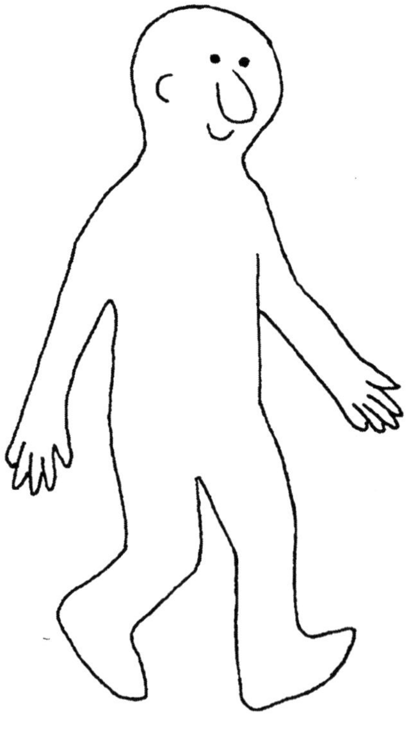

I try to cope with pain by: ______________

____

____

____

Exercise 44

WISH ON A STAR

Purpose:

- Explore feelings about past and present wishes.
- Increase understanding of the needs of others and universality of common concerns.

Materials:

One photocopy of the illustration for each member; pencils and crayons.

Procedure:

1. While materials are handed out, members are asked to think about things they wished for as a child.
2. The leader or a group member reads the poem. Members are asked to share memories about the poem and about childhood wishes.
3. The leader asks members to list three present-day wishes on the blanks. Members may color the picture if they wish.

Group Discussion:

Members share their illustrations and wishes. The leader asks members if they see a difference between their childhood wishes and their present-day wishes. The leader points out common themes expressed in the wishes, such as desires for independence, security, and companionship.

Sharing about common needs in this exercise helps to build a feeling of community and belonging.

Wish on a Star

Star light, Star bright,
First star I see tonight
Wish I may, Wish I might
Have the wish I wish tonight.

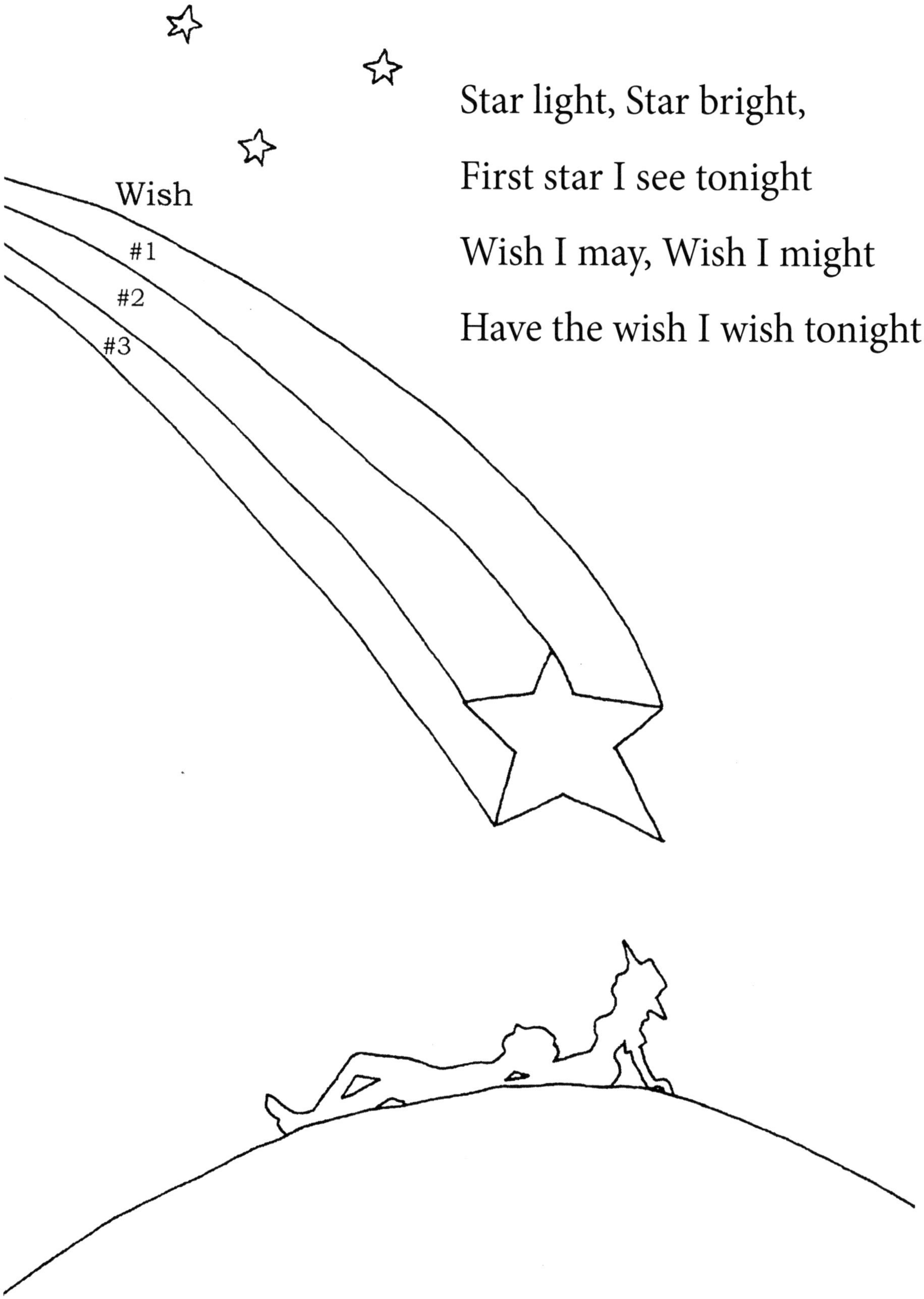

Exercise 45

THANK-YOU CARD

Purpose:

- Develop appreciation for the contributions of others.
- Practice social skill of expressing appreciation.

Materials:

One photocopy of the illustration for each member, folded in half and then folded in half again to form a greeting card; pencils or pens, and fine-line colored felt pens. ***Optional:*** Small pieces of paper and a hat or box.

Procedure:

1. While materials are distributed, the leader explains that the handout is a thank-you card. The leader points out that most people like to feel appreciated, but it is easy to forget to thank others.
2. The members are asked to suggest people in their living situation who might appreciate a thank-you card. Suggestions might include cooks, housekeepers, and gardeners.
3. Members are asked to color flowers on the empty stems and sign their name inside the card. Some members may want to write a message.

Group Discussion:

Members show their cards and tell who they would like to give the card to and why they chose that person. Suggestions are given to members who want to give their card to someone, but don't know how to go about it.

Practicing the social skill of expressing appreciation in a safe environment promotes relatedness and positive interaction.

Variation:

Members may draw each other's names out of a hat or box and give their card to a group member. This variation helps to build group cohesion.

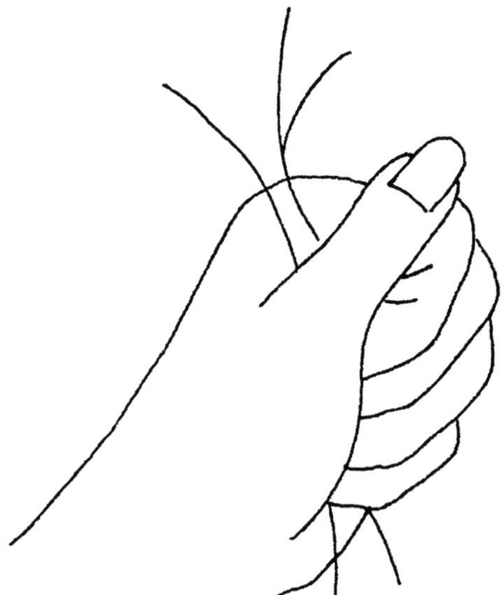

Thank You

Exercise 46

FAMILY BACKGROUNDS

Purpose:

- Promote greater understanding of self and others by sharing family backgrounds.
- Increase trust by practicing self-disclosure in a supportive atmosphere.

Materials:

One photocopy of the illustration for each member; pencils or fine-line colored felt pens.

Procedure:

1. Members are given a photocopy of the picture frame and asked to draw their family. The leader emphasizes that drawing ability is not important. Members who have difficulty drawing may use circles or stick figures to represent family members.
2. The leader explains that a person's position in the family as oldest, youngest, or middle child often affects the role the person plays in the family. The leader gives examples, such as an older child being put in charge of things, or a youngest child being overprotected. Members are asked to think about the role they played in their family.

Group Discussion:

Members show their family drawings and tell about their position in the family as oldest, youngest, or middle child. Each person is asked how family position affected relationships with parents and siblings. Members are asked if their family position still affects how they interact with people.

The leader points out similarities between the families of group members, such as members who were oldest children, or members from large families. Becoming aware of similarities helps to build a sense of belonging and relatedness.

My Family

Exercise 47

WISHING YOU LUCK

Purpose:

- Promote group cohesion by sharing personal information.
- Encourage consideration and awareness of the feelings of others.

Materials:

One photocopy of the illustration for each member, folded in half and then folded in half again to form a greeting card; pens and fine-line colored felt pens; hat or box.

Procedure:

1. While the materials are being distributed, the leader points out that most people have experienced good luck and bad luck sometime in their lives. Members are asked to think about their own experiences of good and bad luck.
2. The leader explains that the folded photocopy is a card to wish someone good luck. Members are told that they will be exchanging cards with each other.
3. Members are instructed to color the card, draw or color something in the pot, and sign their name to the card.
4. Members draw each other's names out of a hat or box and exchange cards with the person whose name they have drawn.

Group Discussion:

Members display the card they have received and reveal which member gave them the card. Members are asked to share about good and bad luck they have experienced in their lives.

Exchanging cards wishing each other good luck encourages feelings of good will and belonging which increases group cohesion.

Variation:

If drawing names from a hat is too confusing for some groups, members can pass their card to a member on their right instead of drawing names.

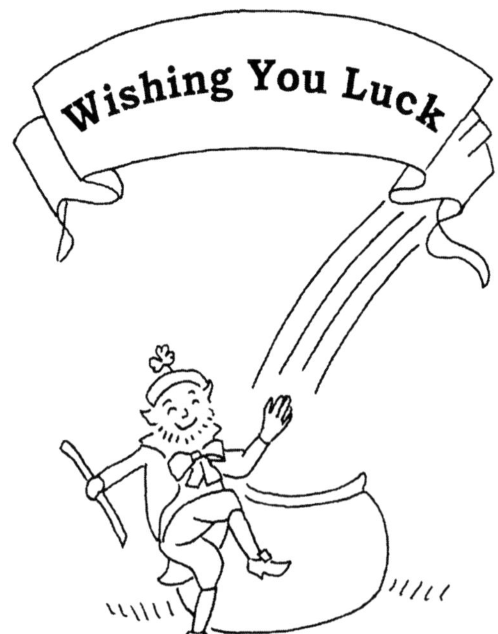
Wishing You Luck

Exercise 48

THE AMERICAN FLAG

Purpose:

- Increase understanding and tolerance of others.
- Promote group cohesion by sharing feelings about a common theme.

Materials:

One photocopy of the illustration for each group member; pencils, crayons, or fine-line colored felt pens. ***Optional:*** large piece of dark blue posterboard; scissors and glue.

Procedure:

1. Materials are handed out. The leader explains that, depending on a person's background, living in the United States has different meanings.
2. The sentence is read aloud. Members are instructed to write their ideas about what living in the United States means to them.
3. Members are asked to add pictures to the flag design of things that remind them of the flag. Members are encouraged to color their pictures.

Group Discussion:

Members share their pictures and ideas about living in the United States. The leader asks if anyone has visited or lived in another country and their reactions to other countries. Members are asked if they have served in the armed forces and how they feel about that experience.

This exercise helps group members to become better acquainted and develop better understanding of each other. Discussions about the flag are especially appropriate around July 4th, Veteran's Day, or Flag Day; however, this exercise can be useful any time of the year.

Variation:

The colored flag designs and other original drawings can be cut out and glued onto dark blue posterboard to form a patriotic poster labeled, "What living in the United States means to me."

The American Flag

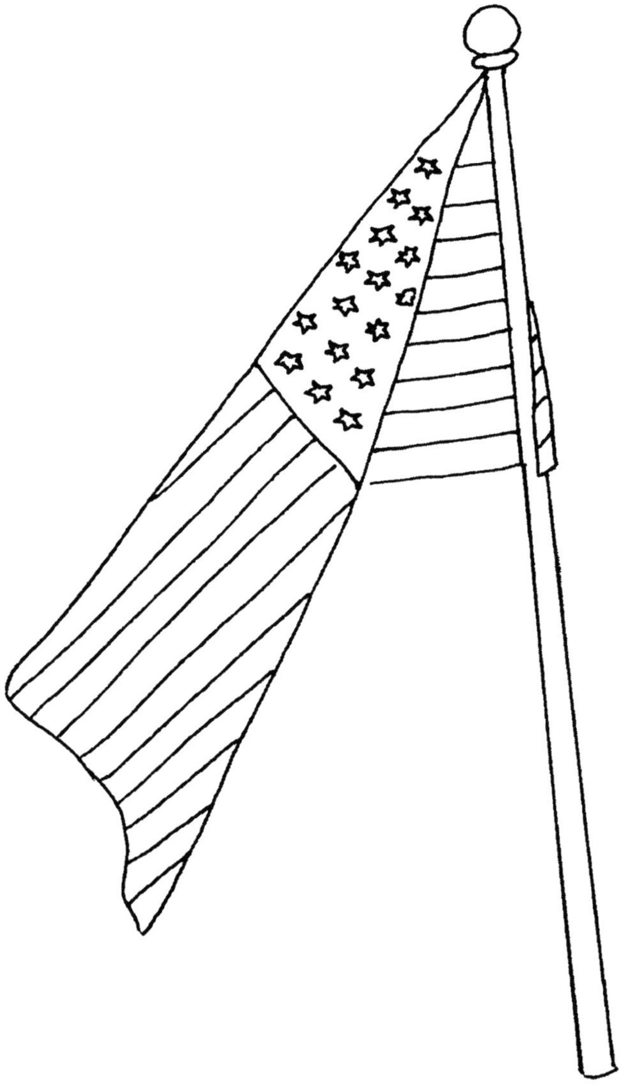

What living in the United States means to me:__________

____

____

____

____

Exercise 49

THE BEST THING SINCE SLICED BREAD

Purpose:

- Promote group cohesiveness by sharing feelings about a common subject in a nonthreatening format.
- Stimulate reminiscence about significant personal history.

Materials:

One photocopy of the illustration for each group member; pencils and crayons.

Procedure:

1. Materials are handed out and the quotation is read aloud. Members are asked if they have heard the saying "The best thing since sliced bread," and what they think the saying means.
2. Members are asked to write down one or more memories involving bread.
3. Members who wish may color the pictures and add drawings of special breads they remember.

Group Discussion:

Members show their pictures and share reminiscence about bread, such as memories of their mother baking bread. Sharing memories about a common, nonthreatening theme helps to build a sense of belonging.

The leader explains that the saying "The best thing since sliced bread" refers to an innovation or invention that is as important as the advent of presliced bread. Members are asked to name something invented since their childhood that they especially appreciate, such as electric dishwashers or television.

This exercise helps to build feelings of belonging since group members may have experiences in common adjusting to innovations and inventions in their lifetimes.

The Best Thing Since Sliced Bread

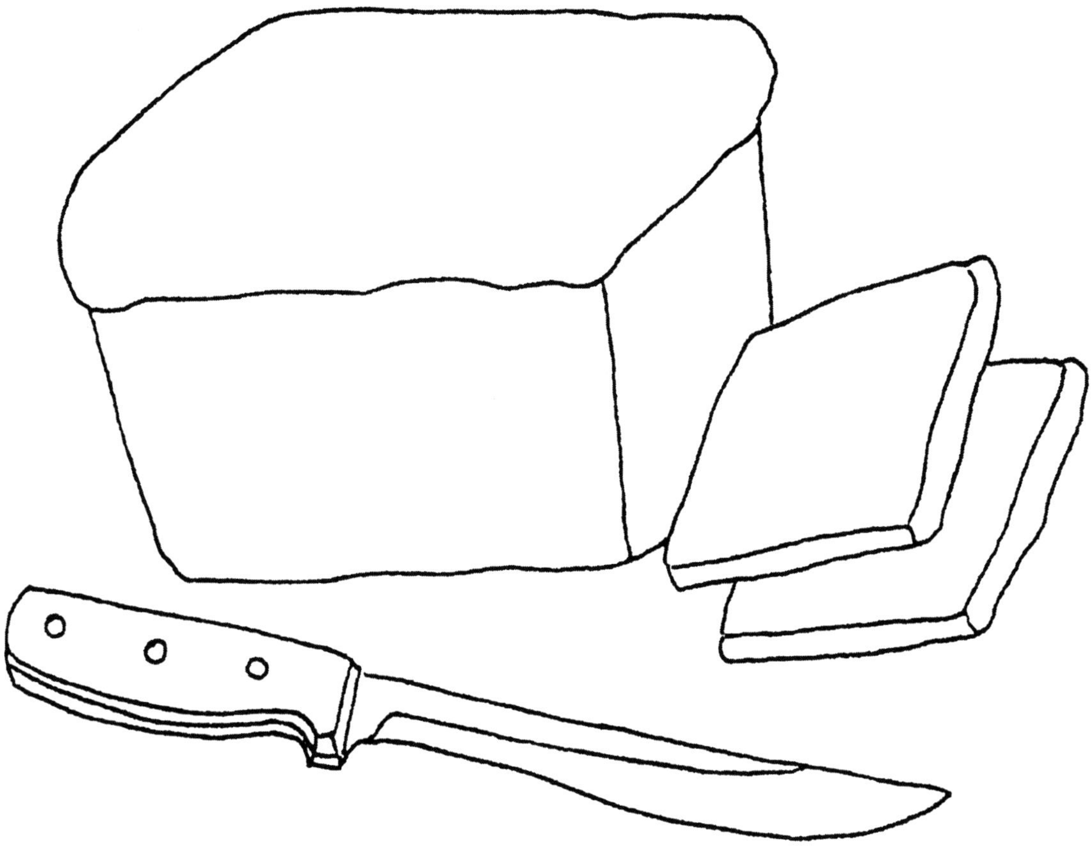

Memories I have about bread: ______________________________

____

____

____

____

Exercise 50

MY HOME STATE

Purpose:

- Enhance identity and self-esteem by sharing personal history.
- Promote interpersonal awareness by increasing knowledge about the backgrounds of others.

Materials:

One photocopy of U.S. map for each group member and one for the leader; pencils and crayons.

Procedure:

1. While materials are handed out, members are asked to think about their home state.
2. The leader explains that growing-up experiences in different states and different parts of the world affect how a person feels about their current living situation.
3. Members are asked to initial and color their home state. If members cannot recall their home state, they can color and initial their present state of residence.

Group Discussion:

One at a time, members share their pictures and information about their home state. Members may reminisce about weather, industries, crops, or seasonal activities of their home state. As each member reveals this information, the group leader fills in a map by writing the member's name on the appropriate state to form a combined map. The combined map is displayed to illustrate which states are represented by various group members.

Members are encouraged to share how they feel about their current state of residence and how they felt about moving from their home state. Members who have lived in the same state all of their lives can share how they feel about this and whether they would have enjoyed living elsewhere.

This exercise helps to increase awareness of others. The leader can emphasize similarities and differences of members' backgrounds to encourage relatedness.

My Home State

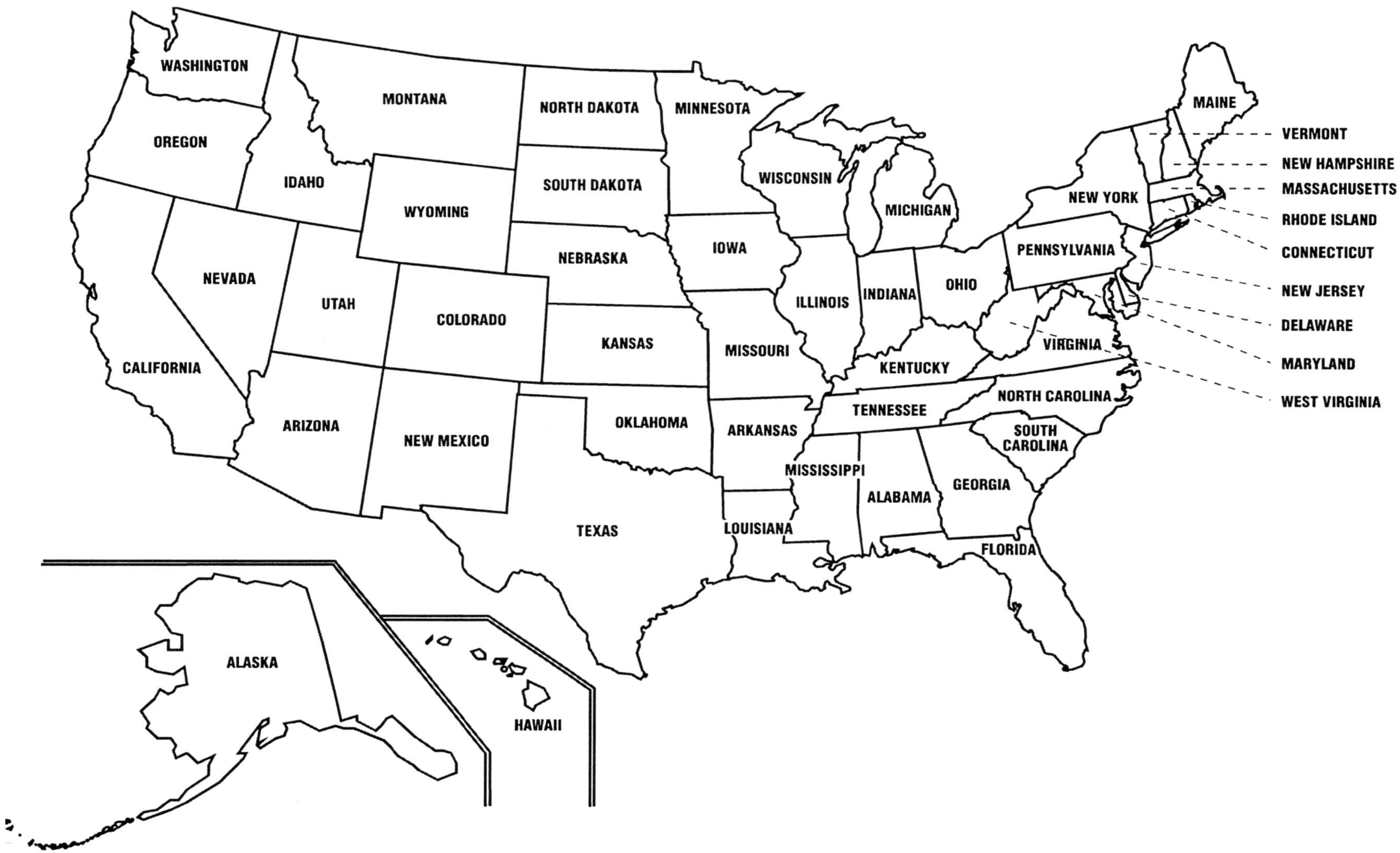

Exercise 51

SETTING BOUNDARIES

Purpose:

- Encourage ventillation of feelings.
- Provide group support in coping effectively.

Materials:

One photocopy of the illustration for each member; pencils and crayons.

Procedure:

1. Materials are distributed and the sentences are read aloud.
2. Members are asked to think about a time when someone intruded on their space and how they felt about this.
3. Members are instructed to complete the sentences. They may color the picture if they wish.

Group Discussion:

Members read their sentences and share feelings about experiences in the past and present when someone has not respected their personal space or possessions. Members are encouraged to describe their feelings and how they coped with intrusions. The leader helps members define appropriate boundaries and develop positive coping techniques.

Older individuals in a group living situation often feel frustrated by the lack of privacy. Sharing feelings in a supportive group setting may help to strengthen coping skills.

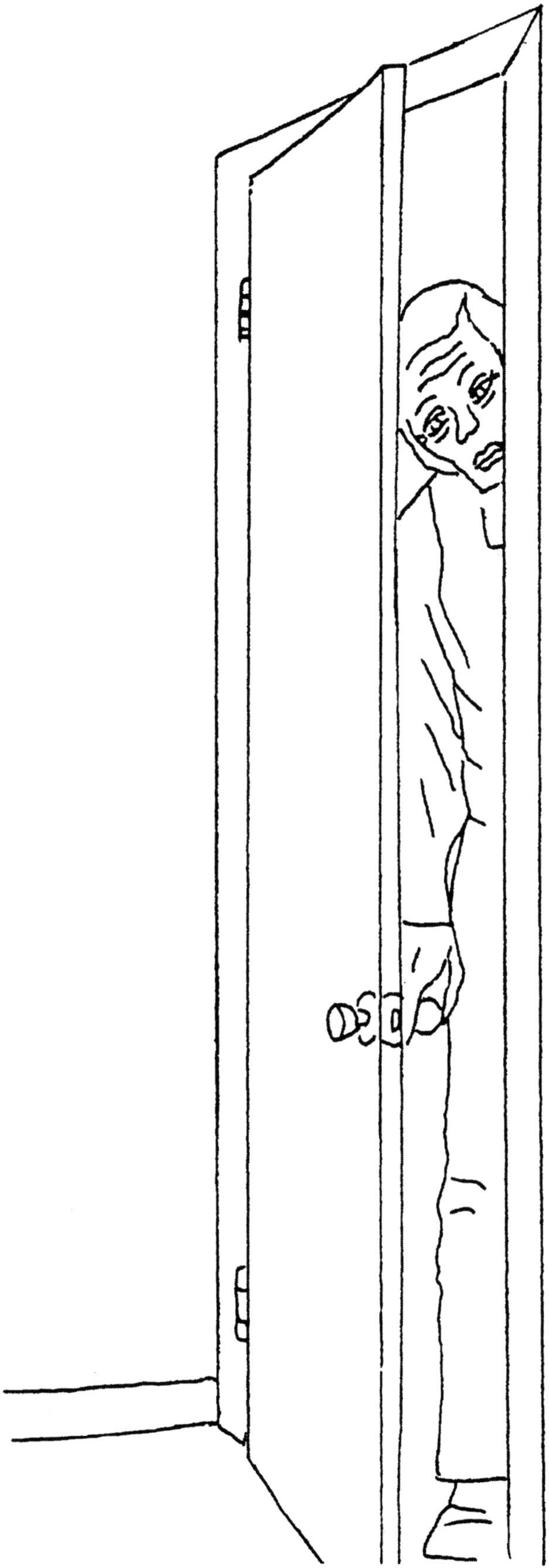

Setting Boundaries

When someone invades my space, I feel: ________

____

____

____

____

____

____

The best way to handle this is to: ____________

____

____

____

____

____

____

Exercise 52

RELAXATION

Purpose:

- Teach techniques to promote relaxation.
- Increase relatedness by sharing personal information.

Materials:

One photocopy of the illustration for each member; pencils and crayons.

Procedure:

1. Group leader explains that relaxation promotes stress reduction and positive coping.
2. Members are given copies of the illustration and asked to write down a relaxing place or draw themselves in a scene they find relaxing. Members may color the scene they prefer.
3. Group members are asked to participate in the following relaxation exercise:

> Clench both hands tightly while I count slowly to 5. 1 . . . 2 . . . 3 . . . 4 . . . 5. Now relax your hands completely. Close your eyes. Take a deep breath. Let the air out slowly. Each time you breathe out, let troubles and worries leave your body. Allow your body to relax completely. Imagine a place that is relaxing for you. Picture the colors and textures. Imagine the small details of this relaxing place. Allow peace and relaxation to permeate your body. Allow yourself to relax more and more. Imagine that you can bring this peaceful feeling with you to any setting by imagining a relaxing scene and reminding yourself to relax . . . relax. Bring this feeling of relaxation with you now back to our group meeting. Slowly open your eyes as I count to 3. 1 . . . 2 . . . 3.

Group Discussion:

Members share about the experience they had during the relaxation exercise. The leader asks for ideas on how to relax. Suggestions might include going to a quiet place, lying down, thinking pleasant thoughts, or taking deep breaths.

Members share their illustrations and tell about a place they think is relaxing. It is important to validate each person's experience during this exercise. Some members may not want to close their eyes and can participate with their eyes open. Some members may not be able to visualize a relaxing place. The leader helps members to focus on a part of the exercise they were able to relate to, such as relaxing the hands by clenching and unclenching or relaxing by taking a deep breath. Members may be able to identify their own relaxation techniques by being asked what they are doing when they feel the most relaxed.

Relaxation

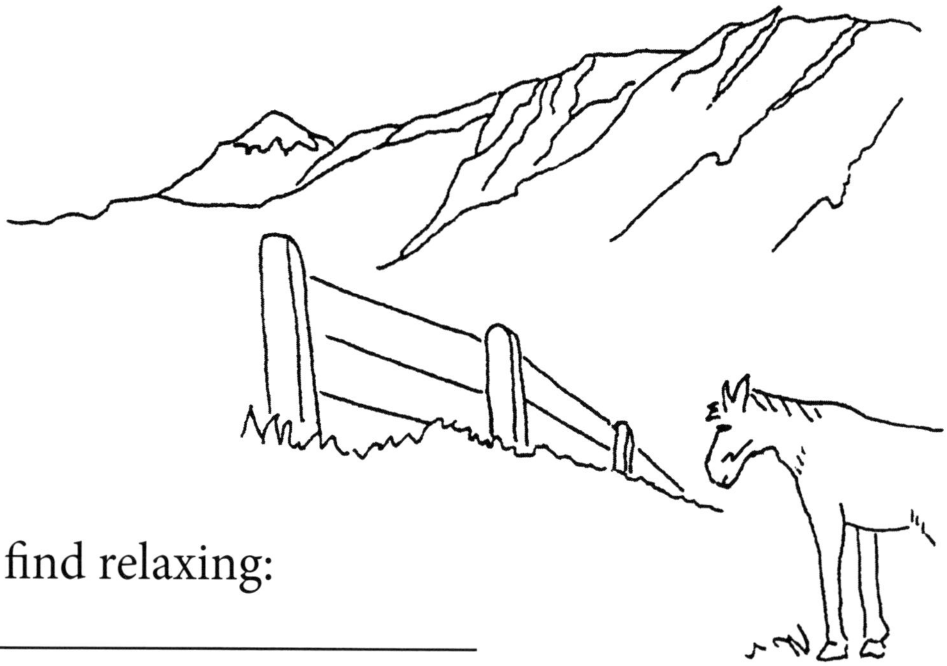

A place I find relaxing:

____

____

____

____

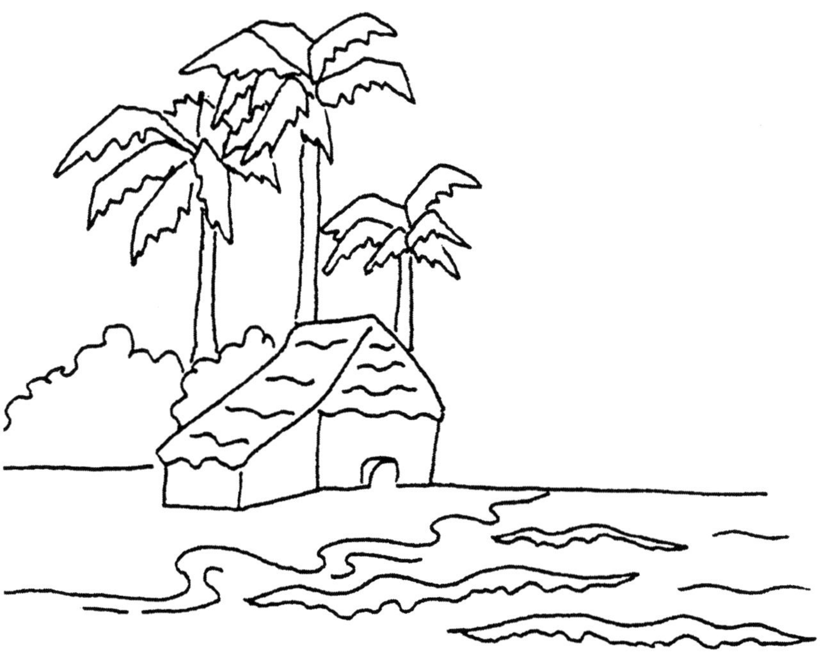

Exercise 53

SURVIVING A HEALTH CRISIS

Purpose:

- Emphasize positive coping skills for survival.
- Promote group cohesiveness by sharing important personal history.

Materials:

One photocopy of the illustration for each group member; pencils, and fine-line colored felt pens or crayons.

Procedure:

1. While materials are passed out, members are asked to think about a time they survived a health crisis.
2. Leader explains that surviving a health crisis makes us not only aware of our vulnerabilities, but also aware of our strengths.
3. Members are asked to draw themselves or someone they know in the hospital scene. If members do not have any experiences with hospitals or ambulances, they are asked to recall some illness they have experienced. Members may color the picture, if they wish.
4. The sentence is read aloud and members are asked to complete the sentences.

Group Discussion:

Members share their illustrations and tell about when they themselves or someone they know survived a health crisis. Members are asked to tell what helped them to survive the crisis.

This exercise helps to promote empathy and understanding for the hardships of others as well as reminding members of strengths they have used to survive.

Surviving a Health Crisis

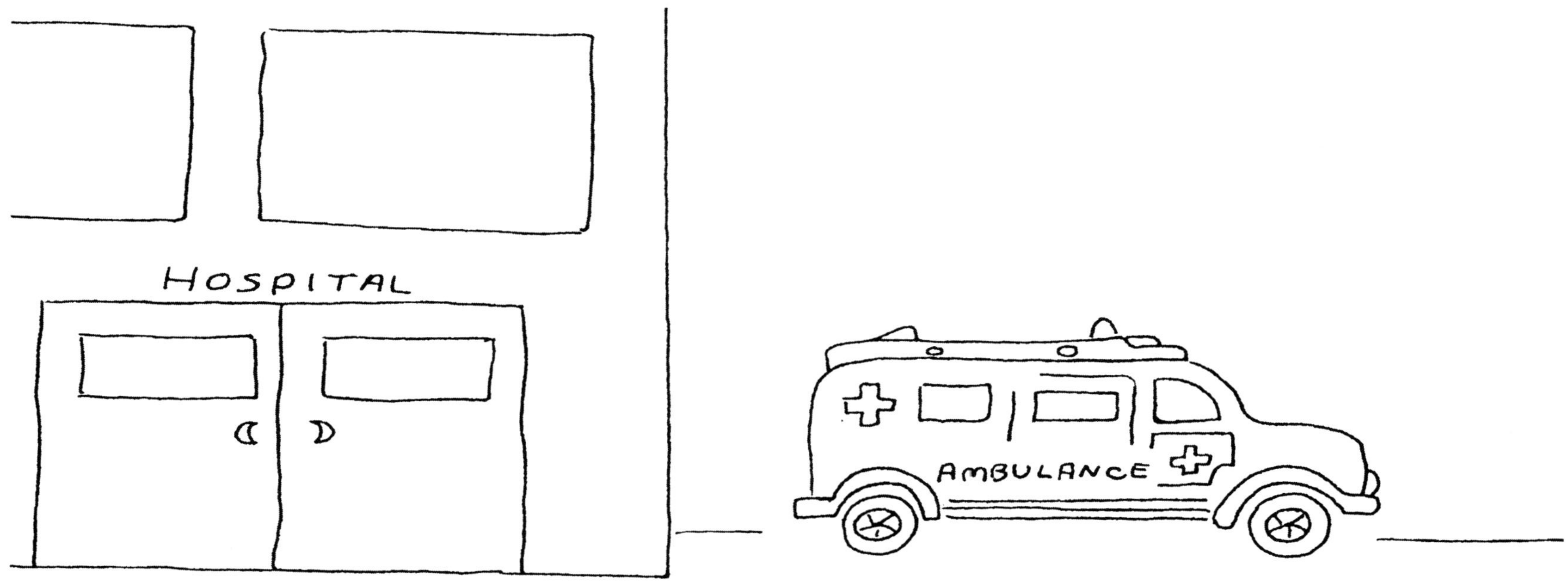

I survived a health crisis when: ______________________________

____

____

I coped by: ______________________________________

____

Exercise 54

TIMEPIECES

Purpose:

- Encourage reminiscence to promote group cohesiveness.
- Practice sharing feelings in a group setting to increase trust and openness.

Materials:

Photocopy of the illustration for each member; pencils and crayons.

Procedure:

1. Materials are distributed.
2. Members are asked to think about associations they have to the various types of clocks pictured. Some members may wish to draw a watch or clock that was special to them. Members may color the drawings if they wish.
3. Members are asked to write in their best and worst times of day.

Group Discussion:

Members share their illustrations and tell about their best and worst times of the day. Members are encouraged to reminisce about the various clocks shown or the clock they have drawn.

Sharing about a common theme that is not highly personal helps members to develop feelings of trust and relatedness. Sharing about worst times of the day can help to open up feelings for group support.

Timepieces

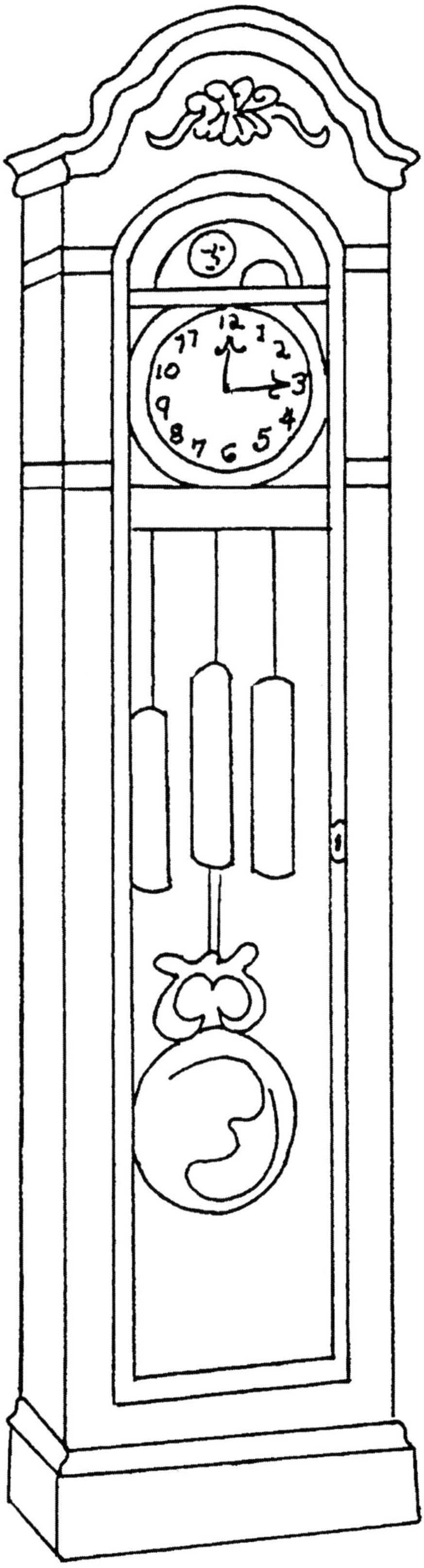

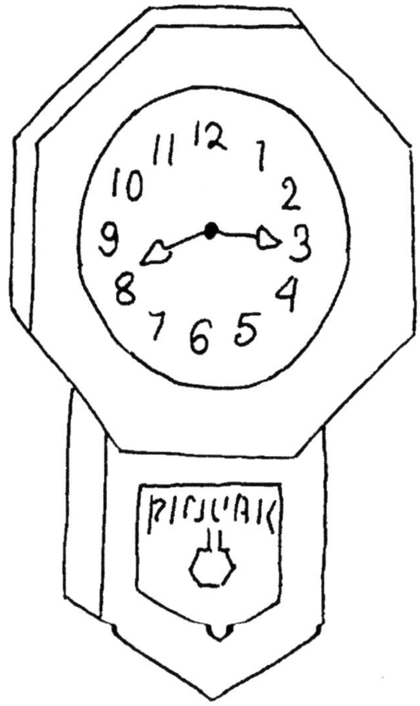

My best time of day: __________

____

____

____

____

My worst time of day: _________

____

____

____

____

Exercise 55

WATCH OUT!

Purpose:

- Share about fears and apprehensions.
- Promote positive coping techniques to deal with fear.

Materials:

One photocopy of the illustration for each member; pencils and crayons.

Procedure:

1. Materials are distributed. The leader asks members what the people in the picture could be seeing and what they might be feeling.
2. Members are asked to write or draw something that could cause the reactions of the people in the picture. Members may color the picture, if they wish.

Group Discussion:

Members share their illustrations and ideas. The leader asks members if they have experienced the feelings depicted in the illustrations. Members are encouraged to tell about specific instances of apprehension or fear. The leader asks members to tell how they would cope with the situations described.

This exercise encourages expression of common fears and worries. Members may feel less isolated with their fears and learn new ways to cope.

Watch Out!

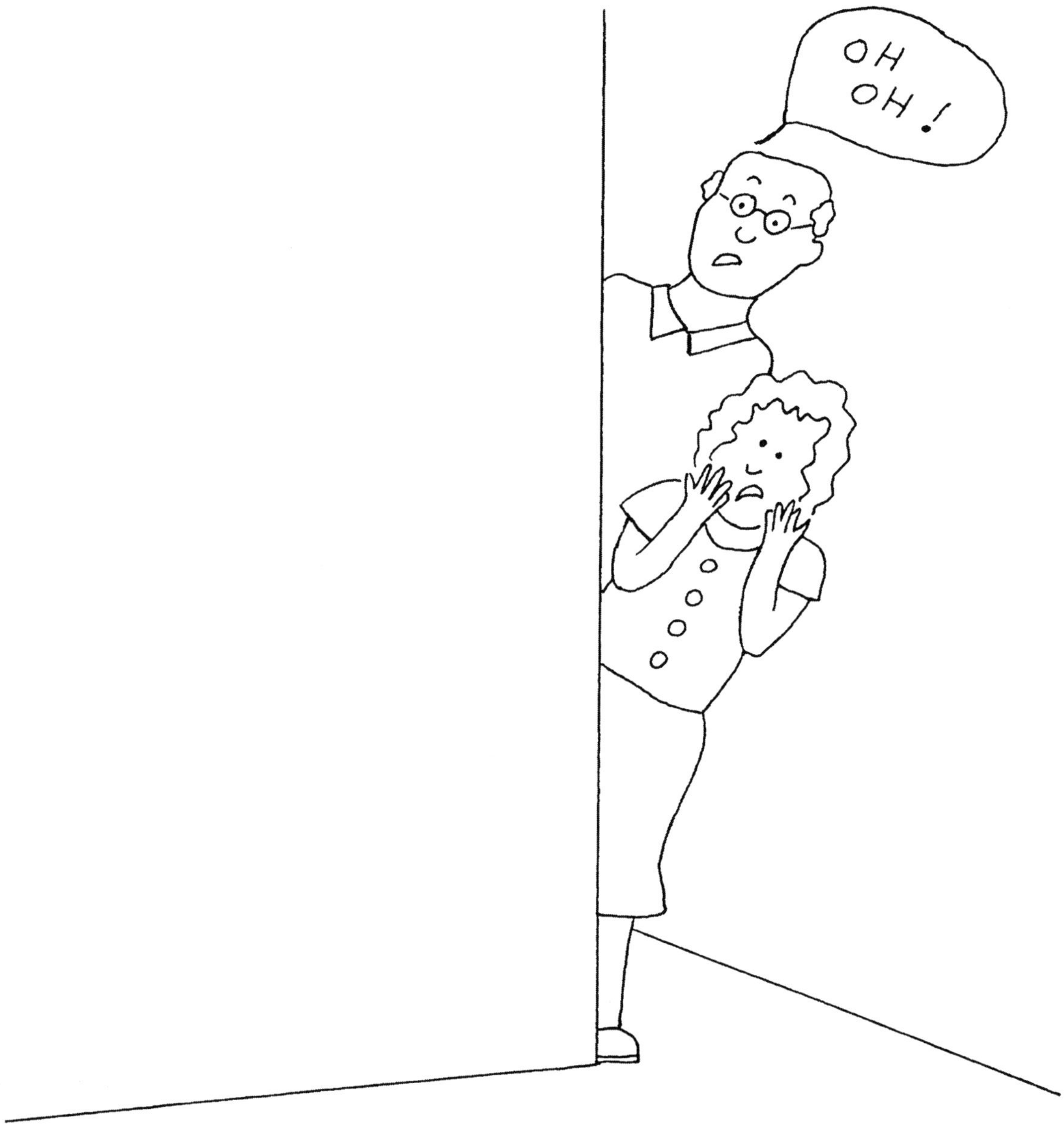

I feel upset when I see: ______________________________

____

____

Exercise 56

LETTING GO

Purpose:

- Allow ventilation of hurts and frustrations.
- Increase empathy and understanding of others.

Materials:

One photocopy of the illustration for each member; pencils and crayons. ***Optional:*** blue posterboard, scissors, and glue.

Procedure:

1. While materials are being handed out, group members are asked to think about old resentments they may have.
2. The leader or a member reads the caption on the photocopy. Members are asked to explain what they think the caption means.
3. Members are asked to list in the blank spaces one or more hurts or resentments they would like to be rid of.
4. Members are encouraged to color the balloon.

Group Discussion:

Members share their illustrations and ideas. Members are asked to tell what makes it hard to let go of their particular resentment, and whether they would feel better if they could get rid of it. The leader asks if anyone in the group can remember getting over a resentment. If any group member can share an example, that person is asked to describe how they accomplished letting go and moving on.

This exercise focuses on one of the important psychological tasks of later life: to work toward resolution of conflicts in order to reduce feelings of worthlessness and despair.

Variation:

The colored balloons can be cut out and glued onto blue posterboard with a copy of the caption as a title.

Letting Go

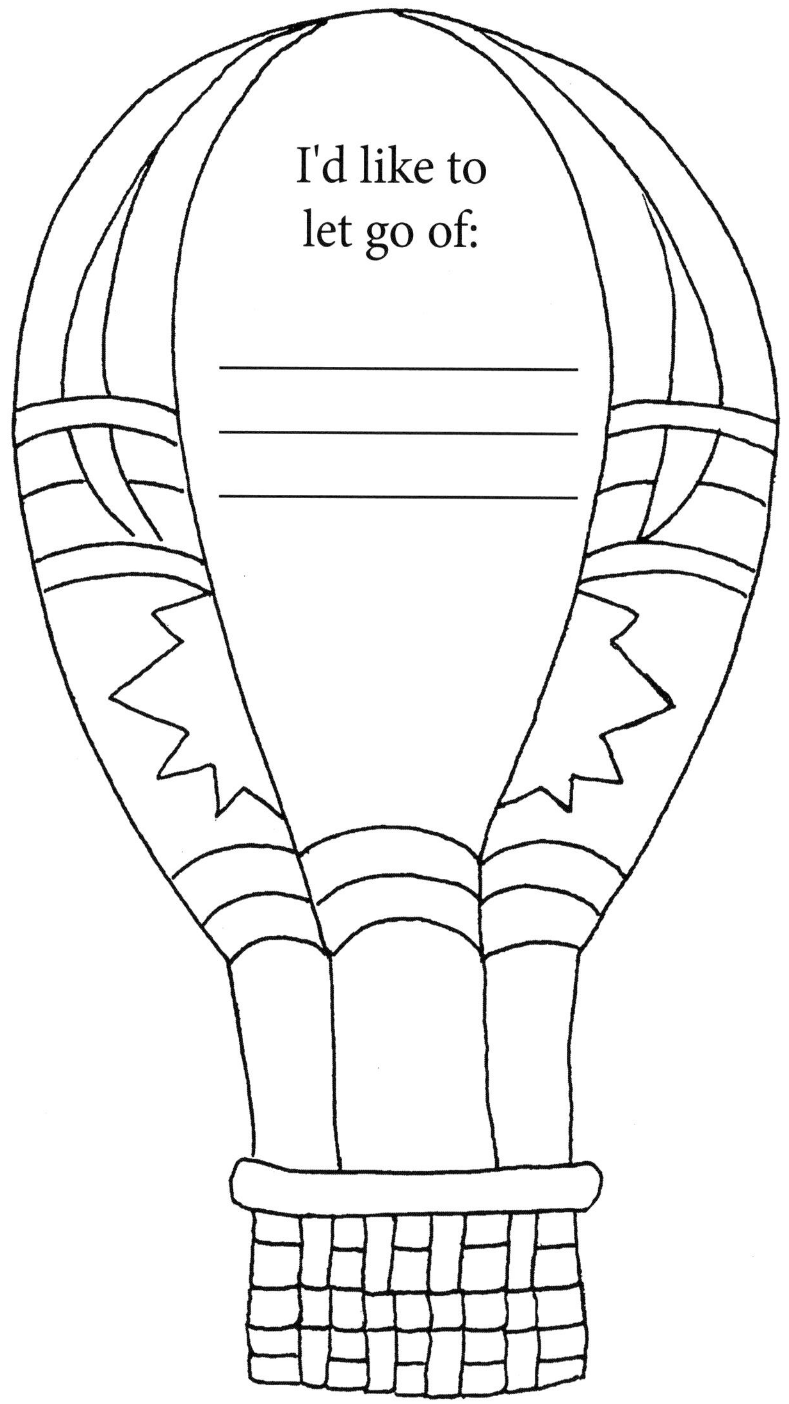

Letting go of resentments lightens the heart
and frees the spirit.

Exercise 57

BLOOM WHERE YOU ARE PLANTED

Purpose:

- Stimulate creative expression and ventilation of feelings.
- Encourage healthy coping skills.

Materials:

One photocopy of the illustration for each group member; crayons or colored felt pens.

Procedure:

1. Materials are distributed. Group members are asked to explain the meaning of the phrase "Bloom where you are planted."
2. Members are instructed to finish the illustration of flowers in the pot and color their picture.

Group Discussion:

Members share their illustrations and tell why a certain flower or color was chosen. The leader clarifies the meaning of the caption by explaining that the saying, "Bloom where you are planted," can mean to make the best of a situation. Members are asked to think of difficult times in their lives when it was hard to make the best of things; for example, a bad work situation or a difficult relationship.

Members are asked to describe how they coped, what helped them to survive, and what they learned from the experience.

Reviewing previous coping skills helps members to stay in touch with personal strengths.

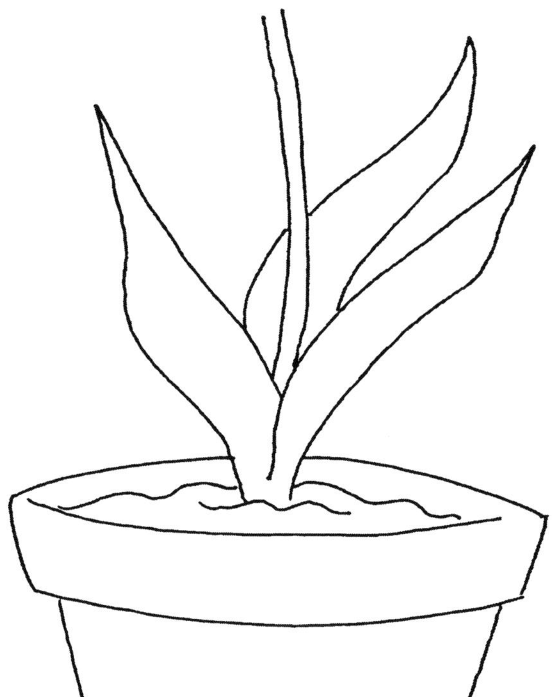

Bloom Where You Are Planted

Exercise 58

MAKING NEW GOALS

Purpose:

- Encourage positive goal formation to instill hope.
- Increase awareness of personal needs.

Materials:

One photocopy of the illustration for each member; pencils and crayons.

Procedure:

1. Materials are passed out and the leader points out that making positive goals is psychologically healthy.
2. Members are asked to think about realistic goals that might improve their life.
3. The statements are read aloud and members are asked to complete the sentences with their goals.
4. Members may color the illustration and draw pictures to represent their goals.

Group Discussion:

Members are asked to share memories and associations triggered by the illustration. The leader asks members to share how they have celebrated the New Year and whether they have made New Year's resolutions.

The leader explains that it is important to make resolutions or set goals throughout the year and throughout life. Members are asked to give examples of realistic, positive goals. Suggestions might include smiling more often, remembering to express appreciation to others, making a new acquaintance, or participating in more activities.

Members share their illustrations and goals. They are asked to explain how they might go about achieving their goals.

This exercise is helpful in stimulating interest in setting realistic goals and raising awareness of remaining areas of choice in the members' lives.

Making New Goals

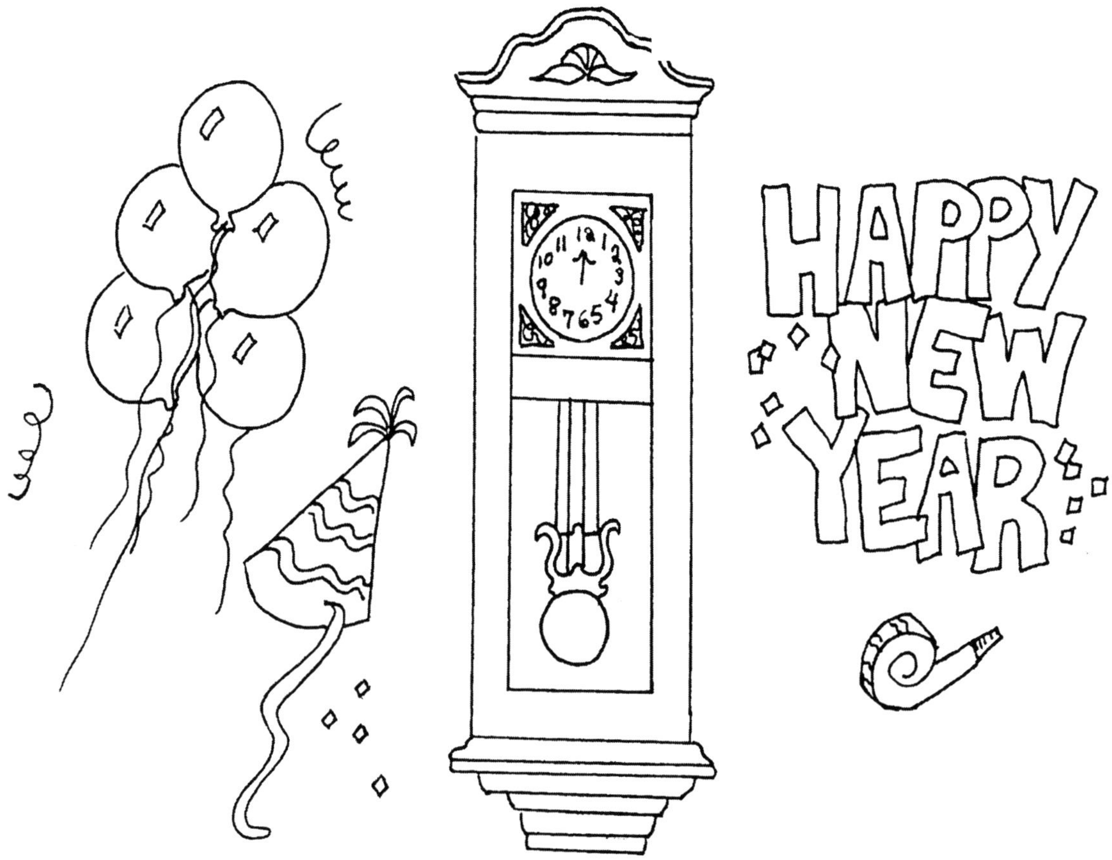

I would like to do more: ______________________________

____

____

I would like to do less: _______________________________

____

____

A goal for next week: _________________________________

____

____

Exercise 59

HELPING EACH OTHER

Purpose:

- Increase self-esteem and feelings of belonging by participation in a group project.
- Emphasize the value of altruistic behavior which enhances positive self-image.

Materials:

Large piece of white posterboard; fine-line colored felt pens. ***Optional:*** a blank sheet of white paper for each member.

Procedure:

1. The leader tells the group that members are going to make a poster together to illustrate helpful attitudes.
2. The leader explains that being helpful is not only beneficial to others but also helps people to feel better about themselves.
3. The group is asked to share ideas on how they can be helpful to others.
4. Each group member selects a colored fine-line felt pen to be used on the poster. It is best to omit yellow because it does not show up well on white posterboard.
5. The leader uses the colored pen chosen by the group member to draw around one hand of the member, placing the palm on the edge of the posterboard with the fingers pointing toward the middle. A large piece of posterboard accomodates 8 to 10 outlines of hands with some overlapping of the fingers.
6. Members are asked to write their names on the outline of their hand in the same color used to draw around the hand.
7. The leader selects a colored felt pen and writes "Helping Hands" in large letters in the middle of the poster.

Group Discussion:

The leader encourages members to tell stories about how they have helped someone in the past or present. Members may also tell about times when they received help. This exercise focuses on positive actions of self and others to increase trust and cooperation.

Variation:

This exercise can be done individually by drawing around members' hands on separate pieces of paper.

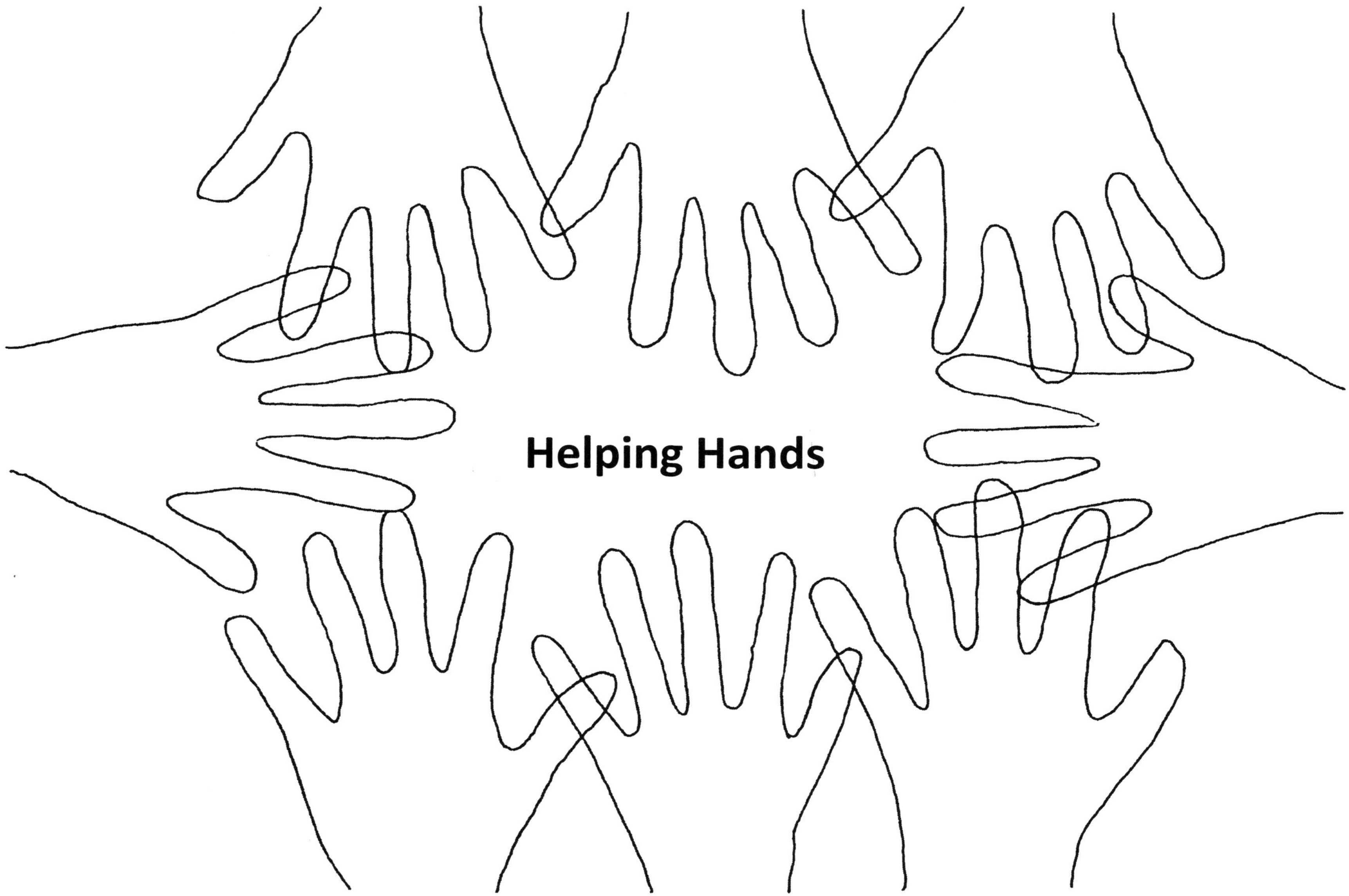
Helping Hands

Exercise 60

MEMORIES OF FATHER

Purpose:

- Increase understanding of self and others by sharing feelings about family.
- Promote resolution of past emotional issues.

Materials:

One photocopy of the illustration for each member; pencils or fine-line colored felt pens.

Procedure:

1. While materials are distributed, group members are asked to think about their father, or a father-figure in their lives. Members are asked to draw a picture of their father and finish the sentences below the picture. Members who did not know their father can draw a person who was father-like.
2. Members share their pictures and sentences.

Group Discussion:

Members share their illustrations and sentences. Validation of feelings is very important in this exercise. Some members may express feelings of loss or unresolved grief about their father. Other members may reveal unpleasant memories or disappointments. In these cases, members can be encouraged to share how they survived and what they did to make up for their fathers' deficits. Members may also be encouraged to tell how their feelings about their father have changed over time.

Memories of Father

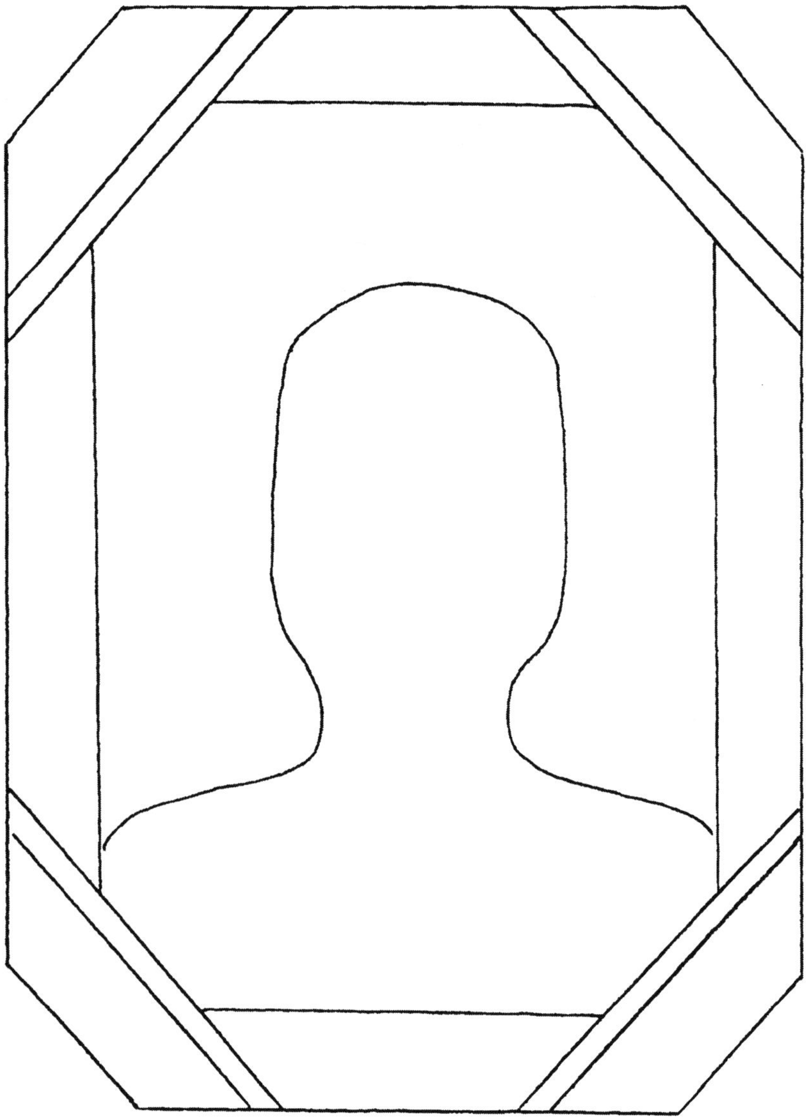

My father was good at: ______________________________

I liked it when he: __________________________________

Sometimes I wished he would: ________________________

If could talk to him today, I'd tell him: ________________

____

Exercise 61

HOW DO YOU FEEL?

Purpose:

- Encourage sharing feelings to promote group empathy and support.
- Relate emotional states to stressors in order to enhance coping abilities.

Materials:

One photocopy of the illustration for each member; pencils.

Procedure:

1. Materials are passed out.
2. Members are asked to guess what feelings are being expressed on the faces at the top of the exercise.
3. The situations under the faces are read out loud. Members are instructed to draw faces that reflect their own feelings in the situations listed. The leader emphasizes that the illustrated faces at the top of the page can be used as examples, but that members are free to draw their own interpretations of expressions on the blank faces.

Group Discussion:

Members display their illustrations and share their feelings about the situations listed. The group leader explains that feelings are neither good nor bad, but that people have choices about how to handle their feelings.

Members are asked for suggestions on how to cope with problematic situations such as those listed. By sharing ideas in a group setting, members may learn new coping strategies.

How Do You Feel?

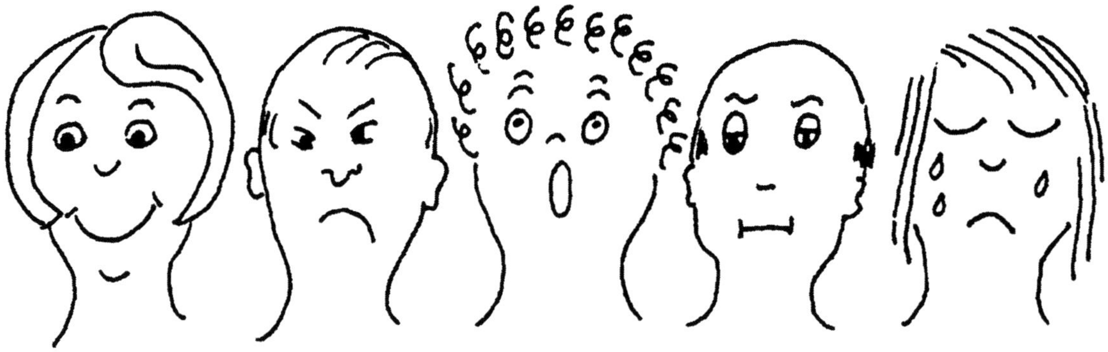

Examples

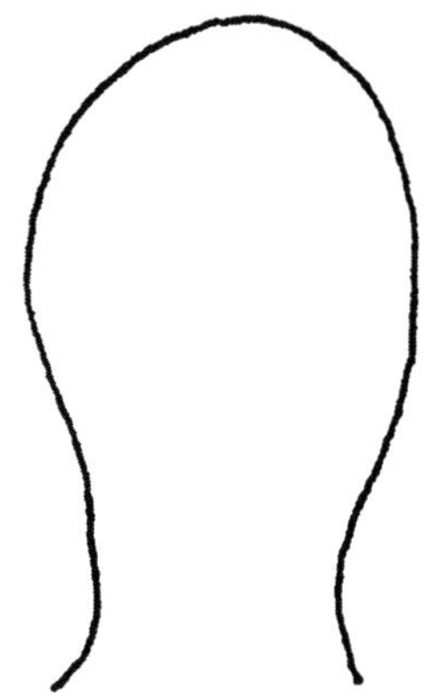

When I
Wake up

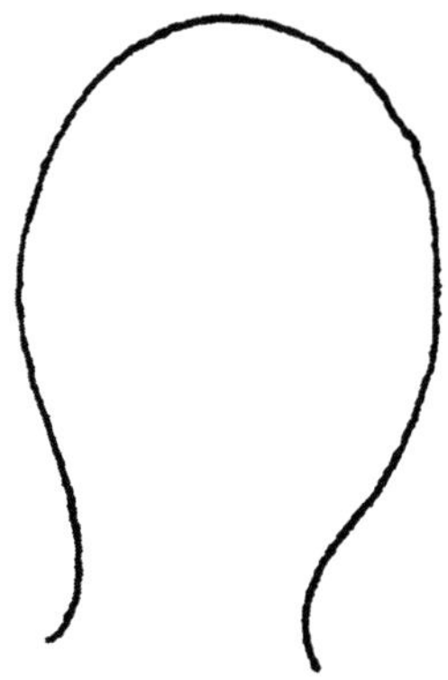

When
Someone Visits

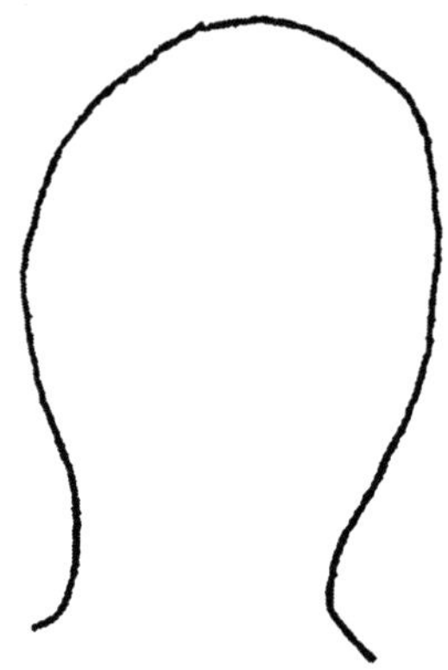

At
Mealtime

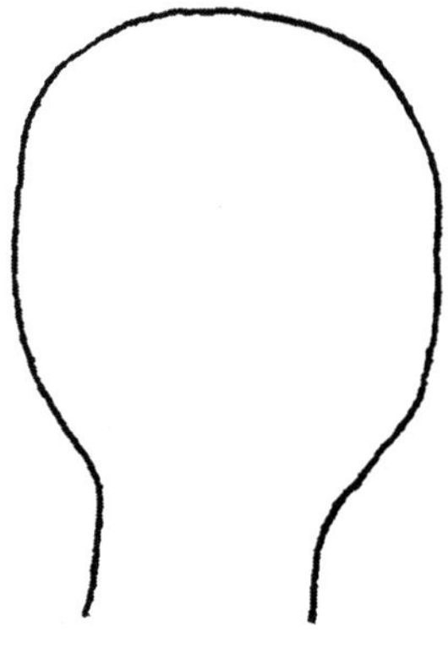

When
People Argue

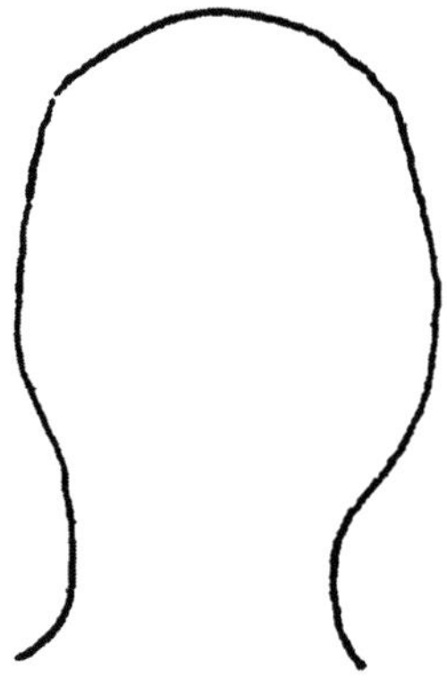

When I
See the Doctor

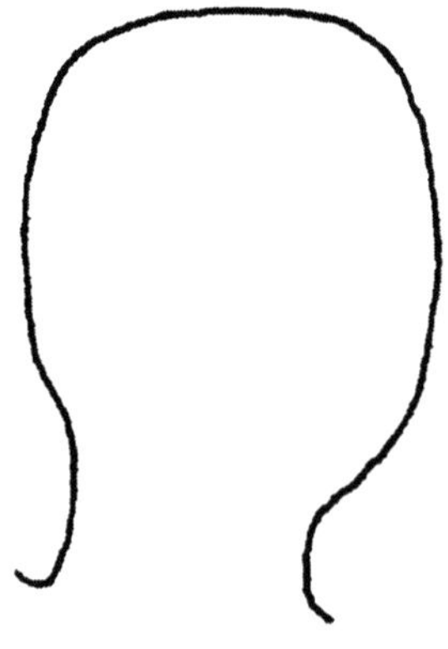

When I
go to Bed

Exercise 62

THE FABLE OF THE TWO GOATS

Purpose:

- Allow ventilation of frustrations regarding self and others.
- Promote positive coping strategies to deal with interpersonal stresses.

Materials:

One photocopy of the illustration for each member; pencils and crayons.

Procedure:

1. The leader explains that fables are stories that are passed from generation to generation because they illustrate truths about people that last over time.
2. Materials are passed out and the leader or a member reads the story (Aesop's Fable) of the two goats out loud.
3. Members are asked to tell what they think the story means.
4. The sentences below the story are read aloud and members are asked to write responses.
5. Members may color the picture if they wish.

Group Discussion:

Members share their illustrations and are asked to tell about stubborn individuals they have encountered in their lives. The leader asks members what they did to cope with the stubborn behavior. The leader validates feelings of frustration expressed by the members and acknowledges the difficulty of altering beliefs and behavior.

Members are asked if they have experienced feeling stubborn themselves about an issue and what led up to this feeling. The leader asks if there is a difference between being stubborn and holding one's ground. The leader points out that holding one's ground can be a beneficial decision if it helps to prevent self-defeating behavior such as alcohol or drug abuse.

The Fable of the Two Goats

Once upon a time two proud goats stared at each other from opposite cliffs of a high mountain range. Between the cliffs lay a deep, rocky valley with a raging river at the bottom. The only bridge across the river was a fallen tree so narrow that only one goat could pass at a time. Both stubborn goats felt they had the right to cross the river first, and each immediately proceeded to walk across the slender log. The two goats met head to head in the middle of the bridge. Neither goat would give way to the other, and, finally, both goats fell headlong into the raging river below.

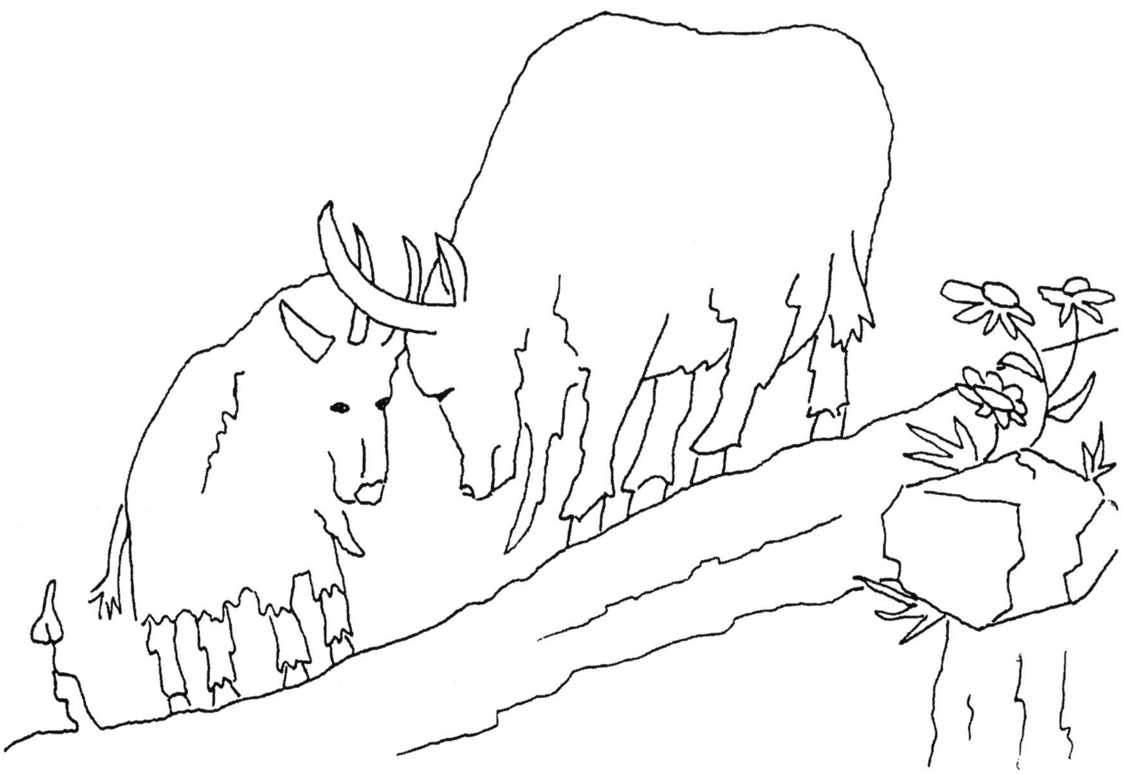

Exercise 63

THINKING AND FEELING

Purpose:

- Raise awareness of how thoughts affect feelings.
- Share feelings to increase group cohesion.

Materials:

One photocopy of the illustration for each member; pencils and fine-line colored felt pens or crayons.

Procedure:

1. Materials are distributed and the leader or a member reads the caption aloud.
2. Members are asked to explain the meaning of "You can't control how other people think and feel, but you can often choose your own thoughts and attitudes."
3. The leader points out that the way you think about a situation affects how you feel about the situation.
4. As an example of how a person's choice of thoughts affects feelings, members are asked to think about annoying dinner partners who may be complaining, rude, or unmannerly. Members are asked how they feel about food when they think about this subject. Members are then asked to think about food at a meal they enjoy; how the food looks and what it tastes like. Members are asked how they feel about these thoughts. The leader points out that how a person feels about dinner is influenced by the kind of thoughts the person is having about the experience.
5. Members are asked to complete the sentences in the illustration and draw a face that shows how the thought makes them feel. Members may draw food on the plate and color the picture if they wish.

Group Discussion:

Members share their illustrations and responses. The leader asks members to share other examples of how thoughts affect feelings. Members are asked to tell about times when it is hard to change one's thoughts. The leader should validate and acknowledge members' feelings. The leader should keep in mind that members who hear voices or have mood disorders may experience times when they cannot choose their thoughts. The leader encourages hope by giving examples of times when the member was able to choose his or her way of thinking. For example, the leader might ask if the member chose to cooperate with bathing this week, or if the member chose to refuse and dwell on how much work it is to get undressed and ready for bath time.

This exercise helps members to realize that they can improve their own mood by choosing to think of unpleasant events in a different way. The idea of changing one's own mood is particularly empowering to elder group members because, in many ways, their choices in life have become very restricted.

Thinking and Feeling

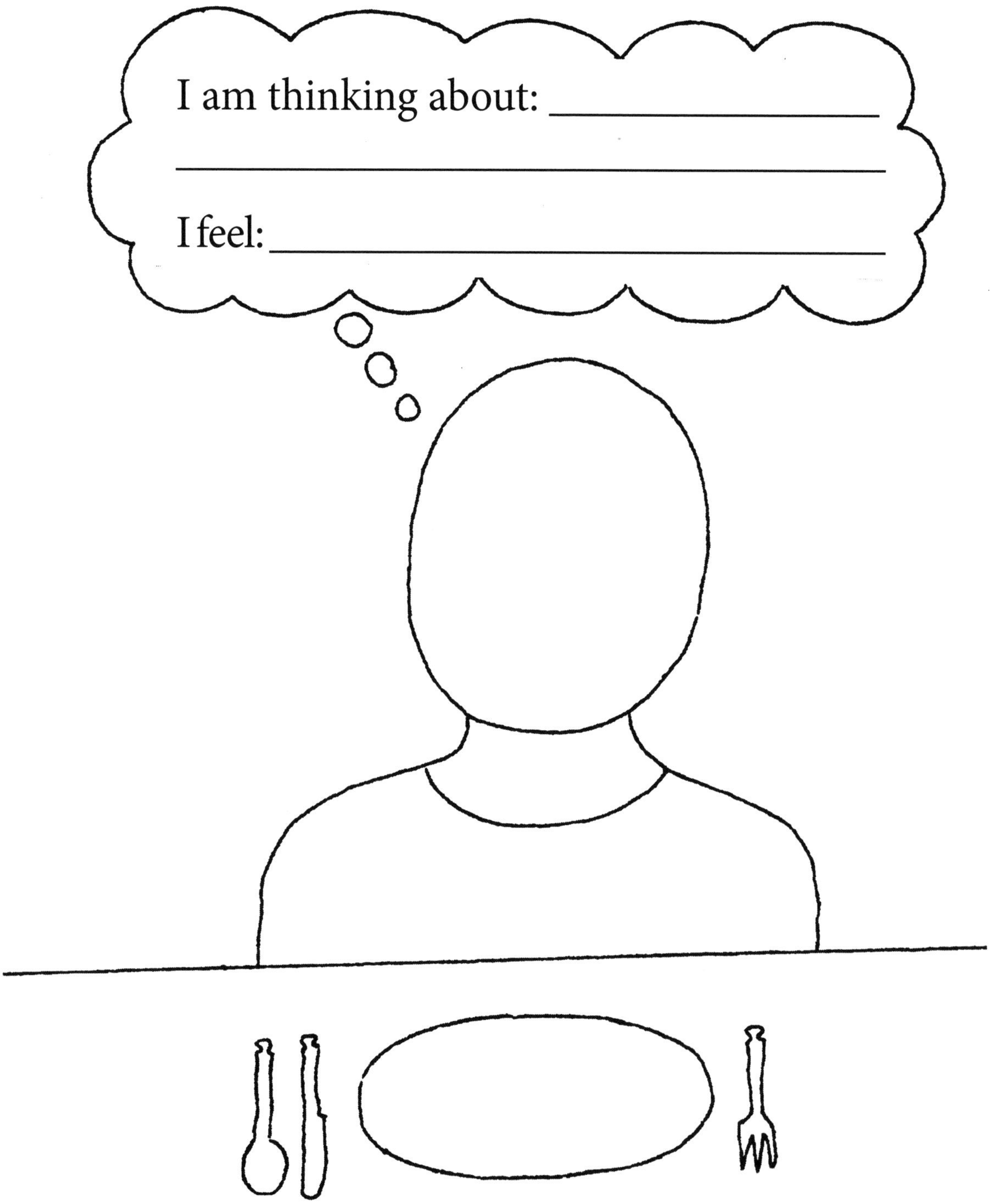

You can't control how other people think and feel,
but you can often choose your own thoughts and attitudes.

Exercise 64

HUMOROUS HALLOWEEN STORY

Purpose:

- Stimulate imagination and sense of humor.
- Promote group cohesion by cooperating in story creation.

Materials:

A pencil and one photocopy of the exercise and story for the leader.

Procedure:

1. The leader explains that the group is going to make up a Halloween story together.
2. The leader goes around the group circle asking for contributions one at a time, filling in the blanks at the top of the Group Leader's Worksheet.
3. The group leader then reads the story on the bottom of the Group Leader's Worksheet, filling in the blanks with the words supplied by the members.

Group Discussion:

Members share their reactions to the story and tell whether they ever played a Halloween trick on someone. Members are asked to share other memories about Halloween, such as experiences of "trick-or-treating" and wearing costumes. Members who did not celebrate Halloween are asked how they felt about not being included.

Most group members enjoy participating in creating a humorous story. Sharing humor helps to increase a sense of well-being and a feeling of belonging.

Group Leader's Worksheet for Humorous Halloween Story

1. A pet: ____________________
2. A vegetable: ____________________
3. Some type of candy: ____________________
4. A reptile: ____________________
5. A spice: ____________________
6. A jungle animal: ____________________
7. A color: ____________________
8. A room in the house: ____________________
9. A farm animal sound: ____________________
10. A piece of furniture: ____________________

- -

THE LITTLE WITCH

One Halloween, the littlest witch decided to play a trick on her pet ____1____. She made a potion out of cold ____2____, gooey ____3____, ground up ____4____, and lots of ____5____. She stirred the potion in a big black pot over the fire. When it was ready, she fed it to her pet ____1____. Her pet ____1____ turned into a ____6____ with ____7____ horns. It chased the little witch all over the ____8____, crying loudly ____9____! ____9____! The little witch hid under the ____10____ and missed Halloween altogether. At midnight, the spell was broken and the little witch's pet returned to normal. She never played a Halloween trick on her pet again.

Exercise 65

HOW DO YOU DO?

Purpose:

- Promote self-disclosure to increase positive sense of self.
- Enhance relatedness by increasing awareness of others.

Materials:

One photocopy of the illustration for each member; pencils, crayons, or fine-line colored felt pens.

Procedure:

1. Materials are distributed and the leader explains that the group is going to do an introduction exercise to get to know each other better.
2. Members are instructed to fill in the blanks on the worksheet. A volunteer is selected to help members who do not write, so that each group member has a completed worksheet.

Group Discussion:

Members share their introductions. After each presentation, the member being introduced selects another group member to ask two questions about the material presented in the introduction. A different member is selected each time so that everyone has an opportunity to ask questions.

This exercise helps to reduce self-absorption and isolation by encouraging interest in others. The exercise enhances identity and encourages good listening skills.

How Do You Do?

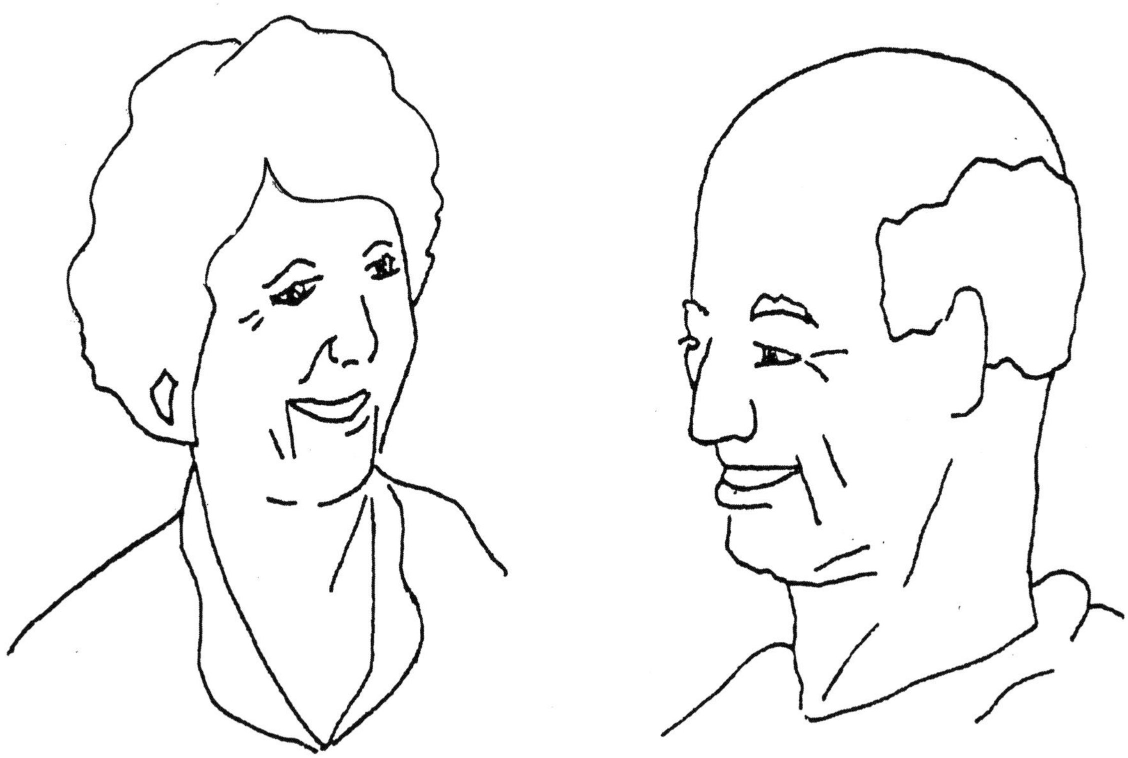

My name is: ________________________________

I grew up in: ________________________________

I enjoy: ________________________________

Today I feel: ________________________________

Exercise 66

TAKE ONE STEP AT A TIME

Purpose:

- Promote positive coping by instilling hope.
- Encourage feelings of belonging by sharing memories.

Materials:

One photocopy of the illustration for each member; crayons or colored felt pens.

Procedure:

1. Materials are passed out and members are asked to explain what they think the saying "Take one step at a time" means.
2. Members are instructed to circle or color footwear that they associate with special memories.
3. Members who wish may draw or color a favorite pair of shoes they have owned.

Group Discussion:

Members share their illustrations and memories about the shoes pictured or other special memories about footwear.

The leader asks members to give specific examples of times in their lives when they have needed to "Take one step at a time." Examples might include taking one step at a time to recover from an illness, make a new friend, or handle a problem.

This exercise encourages a hopeful attitude by reminding members to work on problems gradually beginning with small steps.

Take One Step at a Time

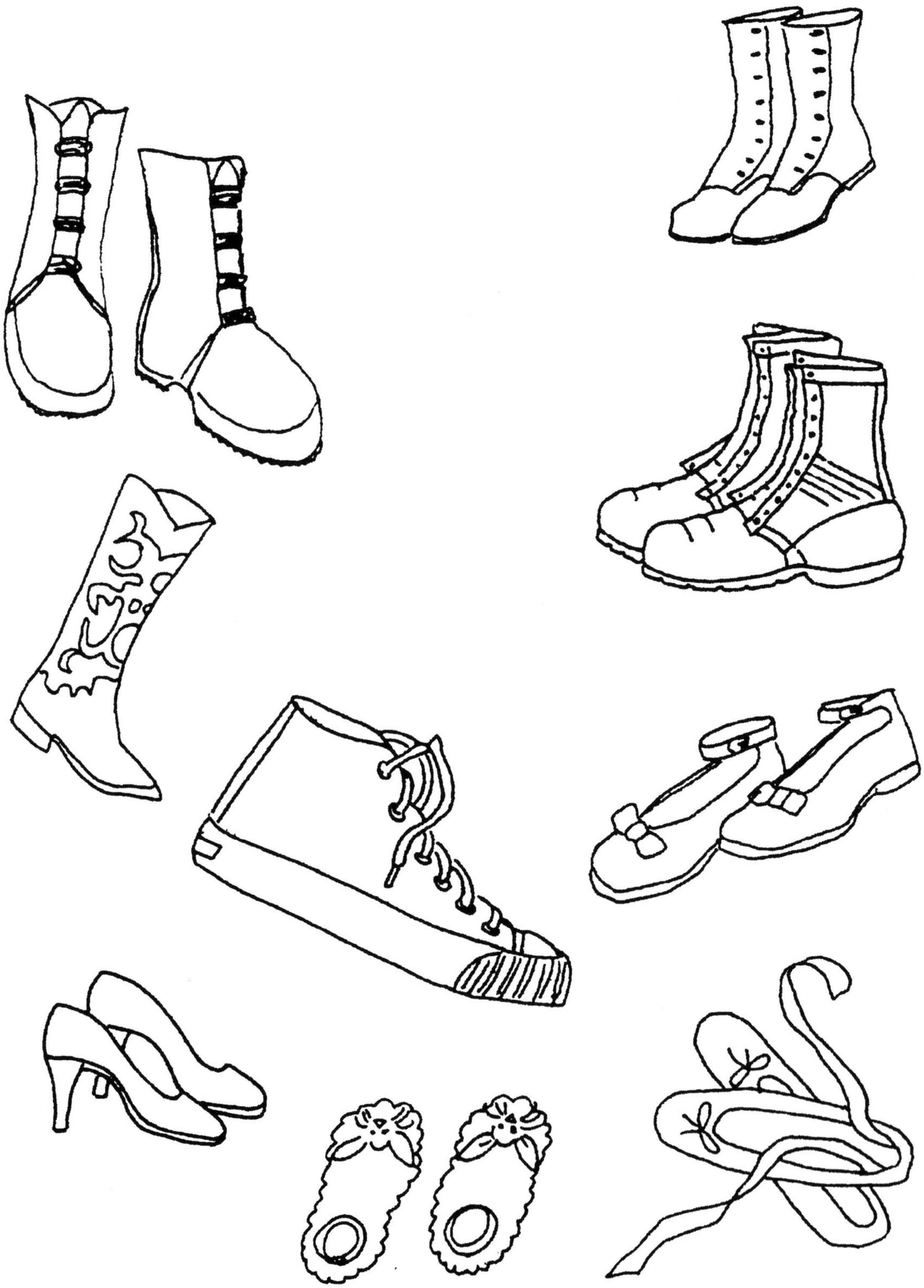

Exercise 67

APPRECIATING DIFFERENCES

Purpose:

- Increase tolerance of differences in others.
- Build feelings of group cohesion and cooperation.

Materials:

Photocopies of wildflowers cut apart so that there is at least one flower for each member; one large sheet of green posterboard; fine-lined colored felt pens; extra blank paper.

Procedure:

1. The leader explains that the group is going to make a poster together to illustrate the topic "Sharing our Similarities and Appreciating our Differences."
2. Members are asked to explain how the topic could apply to people residing in a group living situation.
3. The pictures of the flowers are shown to the group so that each member can choose a picture to color. Some members may want to draw and color their own flower design.
4. The colored pictures are glued onto the posterboard with the topic "Sharing our Similarities and Appreciating our Differences" as a title

Group Discussion:

Members are asked to share memories about the various wildflowers pictured and reactions to the finished poster.

The leader points out that it is often easier to "share similarities" than it is to "appreciate differences." The members are asked what some of the differences are among people in a group living situation that are difficult to handle. The leader may ask members for ideas on coping strategies to deal with frustrations that are expressed.

Members in a group living situation are frequently stressed by close contact with persons very different from themselves. Venting feelings and sharing coping strategies helps members to deal more effectively with the daily stresses of group living.

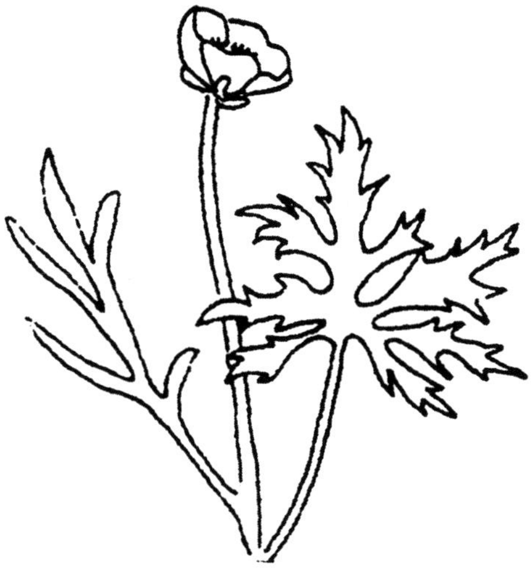

Buttercup

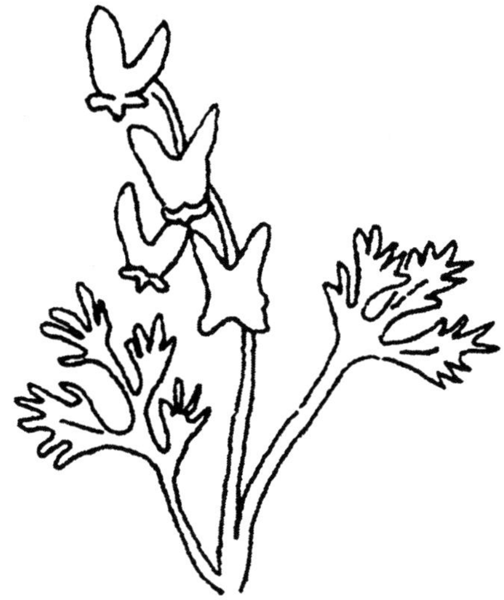

Dutchman's-breeches

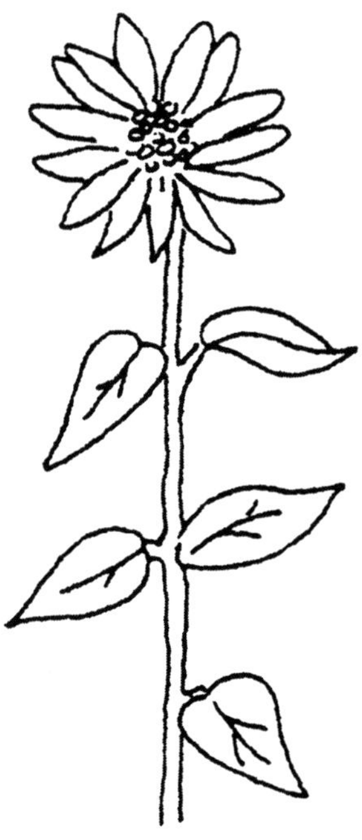

Sunflower

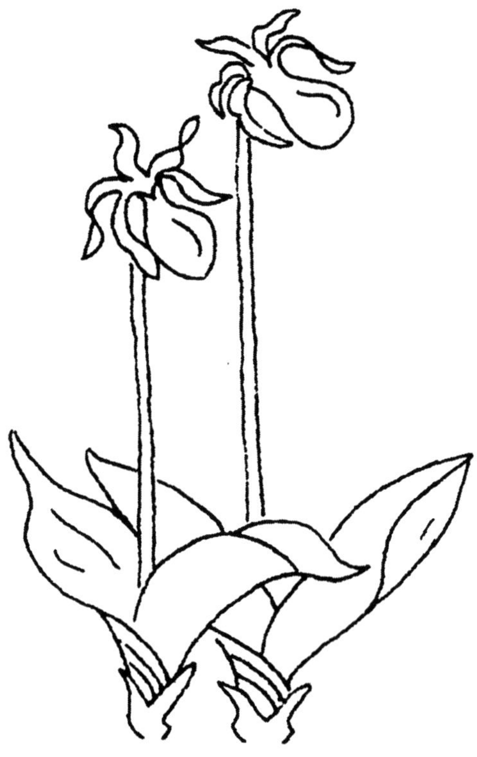

Lady's-slipper

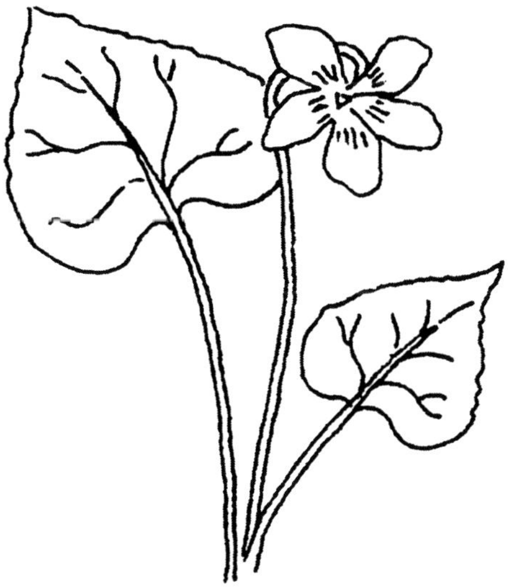

Violet

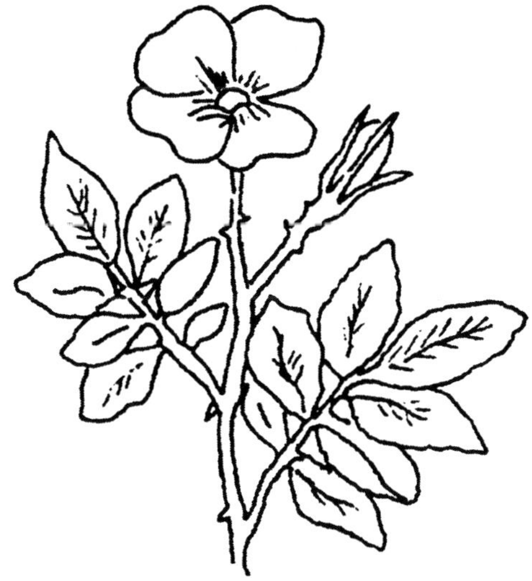

Wild rose

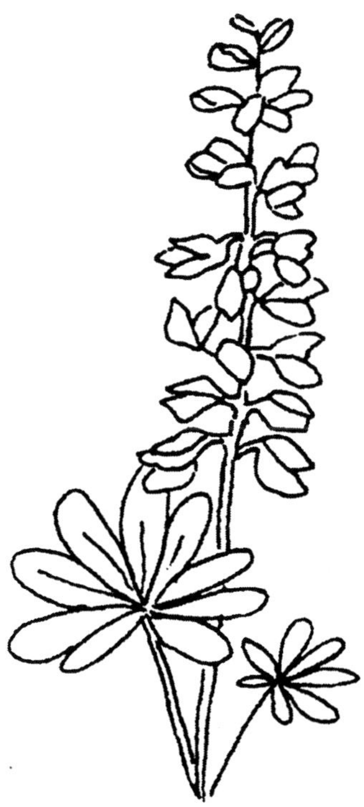

Lupine

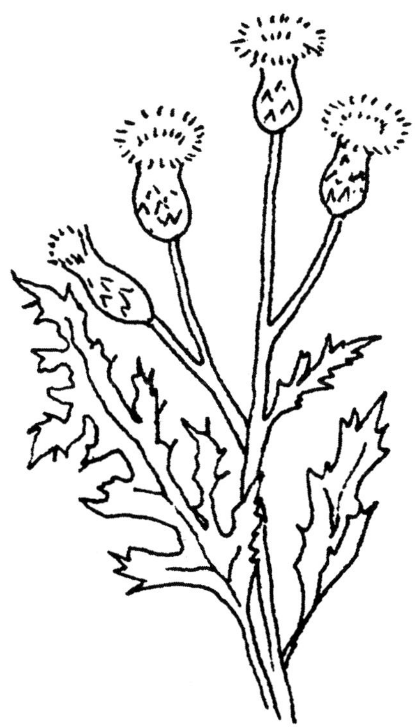

Thistle

Exercise 68

THE BEST THINGS IN LIFE ARE FREE

Purpose:

- Encourage positive ideation.
- Stimulate interest in and appreciation for the environment.

Materials:

One photocopy of the illustration for each member; pencils, colored felt pens, or crayons. ***Optional:*** posterboard, glue, and scissors.

Procedure:

1. While materials are distributed, group members are asked to think of enjoyable things in life that are free.
2. Members are asked to color the picture and add a flower design if they wish.
3. Members are instructed to list things that are enjoyable and free.

Group Discussion:

Members share their illustrations and lists. The leader encourages expression of as many ideas as possible, making special note of ideas accessible to the group members, such as a friendly greeting, a smile, or a hopeful attitude.

This exercise raises group members' awareness of opportunities for enjoyment that don't cost money. Many older group members are on a fixed income and appreciate ideas about mood-enhancing experiences that are free.

Variation:

The butterflies can be cut out and glued onto posterboard with the caption "The Best Things in Life are Free." The ideas suggested by group members can be written between the butterflies with felt pen.

The Best Things in Life are Free

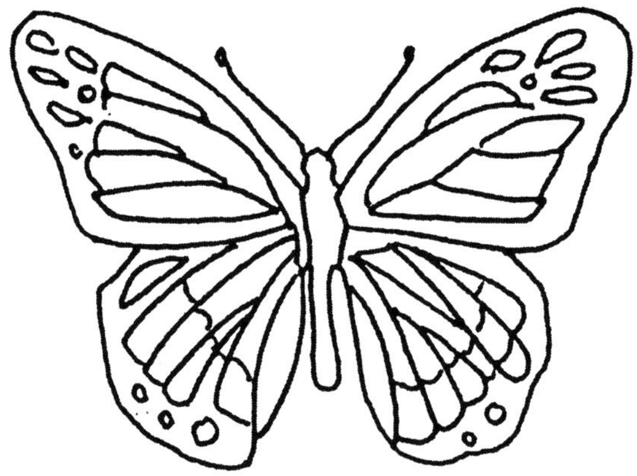

Things I like that are free:

Exercise 69

HOUSE OF FEARS

Purpose:

- Encourage cohesion and relatedness by cooperating on a group project.
- Increase understanding of self and others by sharing memories.

Materials:

One large sheet of orange posterboard, 22" x 28"; one 12" x 18" piece of brown construction paper and one or two 9" x 12" pieces of yellow construction paper; fine-lined black felt pens, scissors, and glue stick.

Procedure:

1. The leader explains that the group is going to make a poster of a haunted house.
2. Group leader cuts 2" x 6" triangles out of the top corners of the brown paper to form a roof line for a house (see illustration of house on next page). The leader folds a 9" x 12" piece of yellow construction paper into eighths and cuts on the folds to form eight rectangles for windows and a door.
3. Each group member is given one of the small yellow rectangles and asked to draw a Halloween design on it with a black felt pen. Members who like to draw are asked to help members who do not draw. Suggestions for designs might include pumpkins, ghosts, witches, skeletons, and so forth. One rectangle is chosen for the front door.
4. The leader glues the brown house onto the orange posterboard and glues on the "windows" and "door." Black grill-work on the rooftop and a few bats in the sky can be added with black felt pens. The poster is labelled "House of Fears" with a black felt pen.

Group Discussion:

Members are asked to share Halloween memories and fears. The leader asks if members ever thought a house was haunted and whether they believe in ghosts, or whether they were afraid of the dark.

Members share feelings and reactions to seeing their artwork combined into a group poster.

Contributing to a creative group project enhances a sense of belonging and increases self-esteem. Sharing childhood fears and fantasies promotes group cohesion.

Variation:

Each member is given a copy of the illustration and asked to draw or write fears in the window spaces.

House of Fears

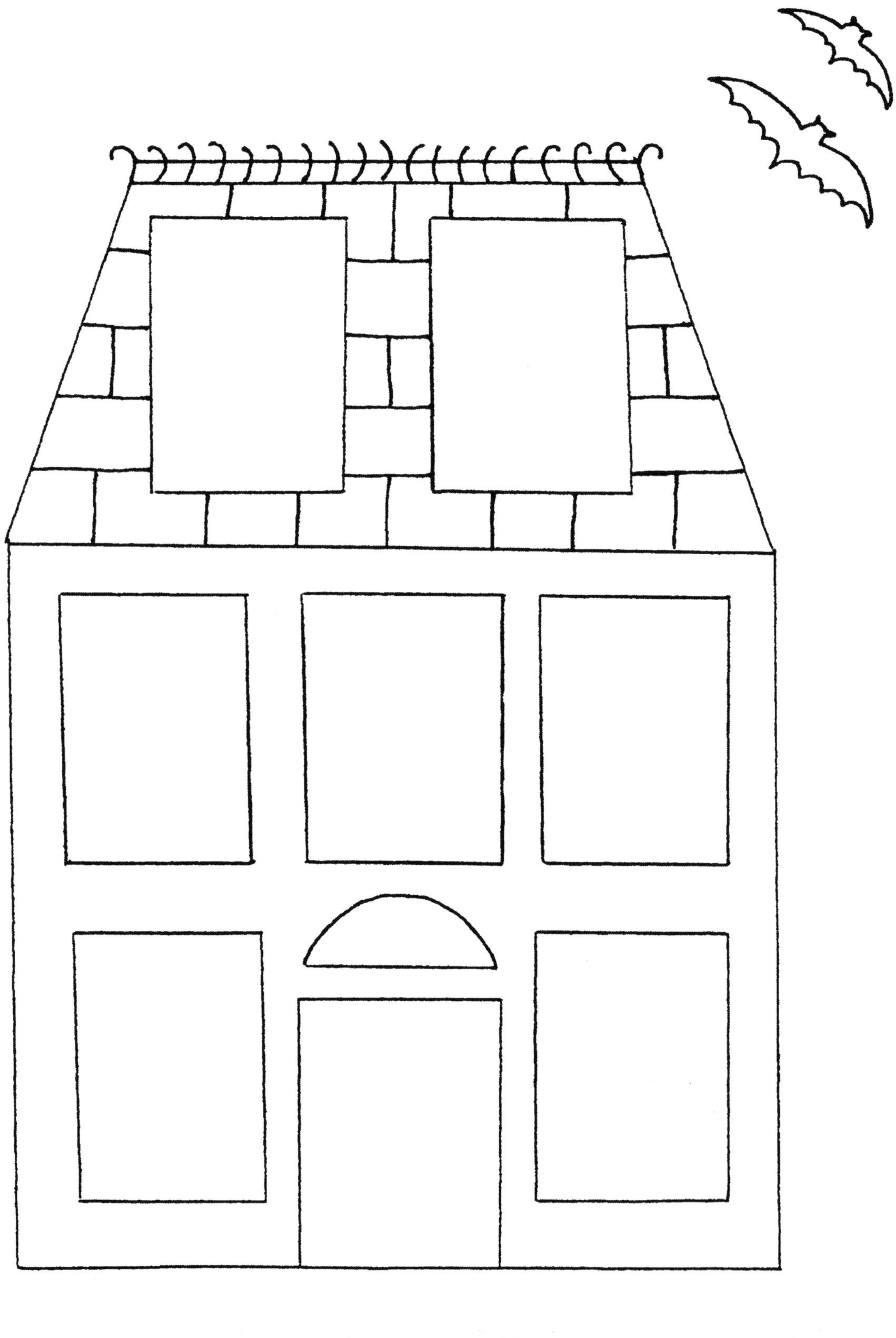

Exercise 70

THANKSGIVING CARDS

Purpose:

- Increase awareness of the feelings of others.
- Build feelings of community and group cohesion.

Materials:

One photocopy of the illustration for each group member; fine-line colored felt pens; small slips of paper and a hat or box.

Procedure:

1. While materials are being passed out, the leader explains that the photocopy is a Thanksgiving card.
2. Members are instructed to fold the photocopy in half and then in half again to form a card.
3. The leader writes each member's name on a small piece of paper and puts the name in a hat.
4. Each member draws a name from the hat and writes this name on the card.
5. Members are asked to identify the pictures on the front and back of the card. The leader points out that the food items on the back of the card are often pictured in cornucopias.
6. Members are encouraged to draw and color items in the cornucopia to complete the picture.
7. Members are asked to sign their name inside the card. They may also write a Thanksgiving message if they wish.

Group Discussion:

Members exchange cards and share the card they received, displaying the card and telling who gave them the card. Members share feelings and reactions to making and receiving handmade cards. The leader points out that it is not always necessary to buy an expensive card to convey a thoughtful message.

This group exercise is helpful in building feelings of belonging and inclusion.

Happy Thanksgiving

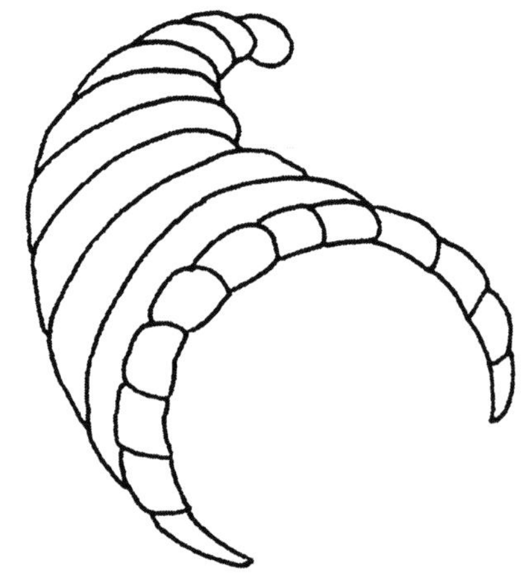

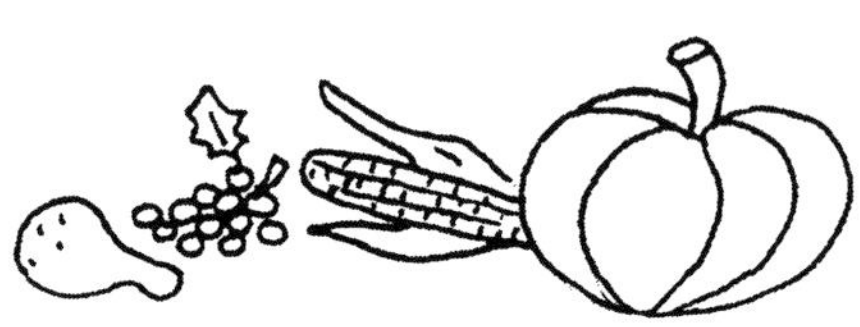

Exercise 71

CHANGES IN OUR LIVES

Purpose:

- Share feelings about changes in life.
- Encourage positive attitudes about change.

Materials:

One photocopy of the illustration for each member; fine-line colored felt pens. ***Optional:*** posterboard to make a group collage.

Procedure:

1. As materials are distributed, members are asked to think about changes in their lives.
2. The leader or a group member reads the caption on the photocopy. Members are asked to explain what they think the saying means.
3. Members are asked to color fall leaves on the trees to represent changes in nature.

Group Discussion:

The leader explains that many people resist change because they are afraid of the unknown, but changes can sometimes lead to new opportunities such as losing a job and finding a better one or moving to a different location and meeting new friends. Members are asked to tell about changes in their lives that have led to new opportunities. Discussion topics might include moving to a new place, changing jobs, improvements in health care, or changes in family structure. Members are asked to tell about attitudes that help a person adapt to change, such as flexibility, open-mindedness, and willingness to try new experiences.

Many changes in life are unavoidable. Sharing feelings about change and ways to adjust to new circumstances helps members to strengthen their abilities to cope with changes in their lives.

Variation:

A group poster can be made by cutting a rectangle around each tree to remove excess border and glueing the tree designs to colored poster board. A copy of the caption can be used as a title for the poster.

Members often experience pride and increased self-esteem from seeing their artwork combined into a group poster.

Changes in Our Lives

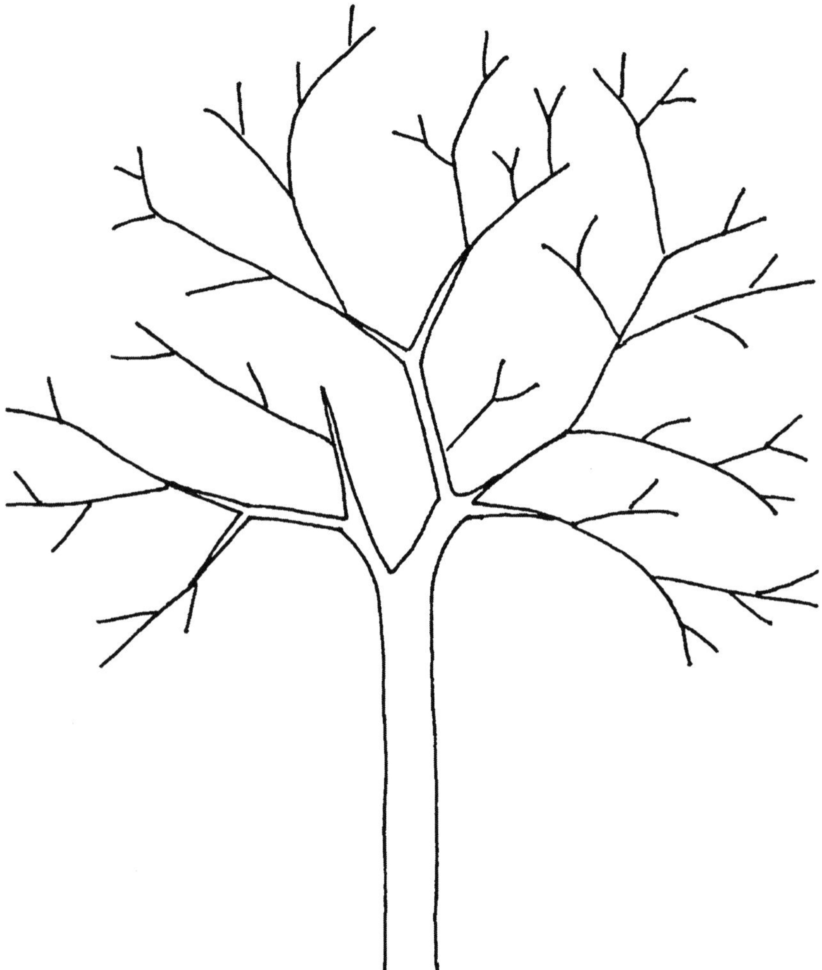

Changes in our lives
Like changes in the seasons
Bring new challenges
And opportunities for growth.

Exercise 72

LET'S PRESERVE

Purpose:

- Increase relatedness by sharing memories in a nonthreatening format.
- Stimulate positive cognition and goal formation.

Materials:

One photocopy of the illustration for each member; crayons and pencils.

Procedure:

1. Materials are passed out and group members are encouraged to share memories of canning, preserving, or other methods of food preservation.
2. Members are asked to describe the contents of the first jar and fill in the label if they wish.
3. The leader points out that the idea of preserving can be applied to saving the environment. Members are asked to give ideas regarding natural resources that need preservation efforts.
4. Members are asked to write in or draw and color items for preserving in the empty jars. Drawings may depict actual food items or environmental concerns. Other ideas can be listed on the blank lines.

Group Discussion:

Members share their illustrations and ideas. Members are asked to share memories of canning and food preservation. Topics of discussion might include pickeling, use of smokehouses, and fruit cellars.

Members are encouraged to explore whether their residence supports recycling efforts and find out ways they can help.

This exercise encourages reminiscence as well as stimulating interest in current topics of concern about environmental issues. Encouraging interest in current affairs helps to increase motivation and interest in living.

Let's Preserve

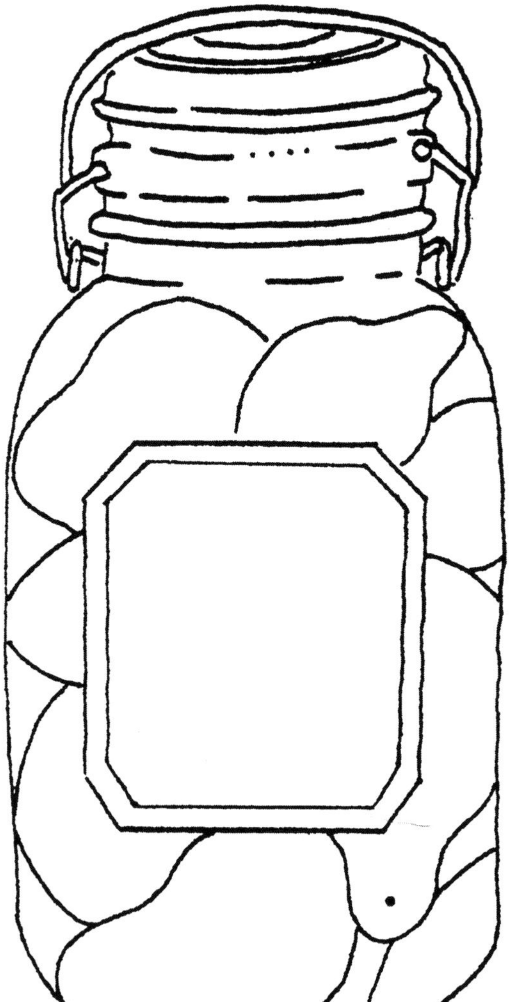

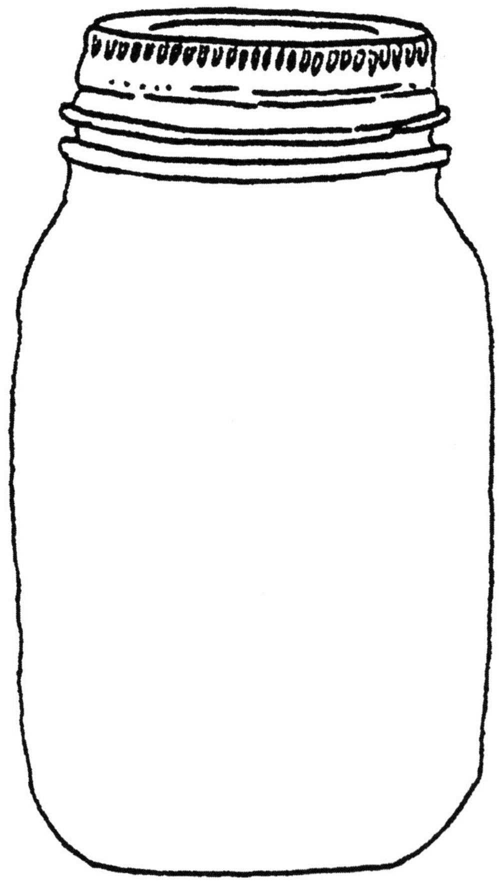

Exercise 73

COW KNOW-HOW

Purpose:

- Share positive coping skills in a humorous, nonthreatening format.
- Promote self-disclosure and greater awareness of others.

Materials:

One photocopy of the illustration for each group member; pencils and crayons.

Procedure:

1. Materials are distributed.
2. Members go around the circle taking turns reading lines in the "Cow Know-How" worksheet.
3. Members check boxes opposite statements that have been addressed to themselves or others in their childhood.
4. Members may color the picture if they wish and add other farm details to the picture.

Group Discussion:

Members share their illustrations and tell why they checked certain statements. The leader explains that early family messages affect a person's self-image. Members discuss which sayings are helpful and which should be replaced with more positive self-statements.

Members are asked to add to the list other negative or positive messages from childhood that had an impact on their self-image.

This exercise encourages self-revelation and opens the participants to feedback which may help to form a more positive self-image.

Cow Know-How

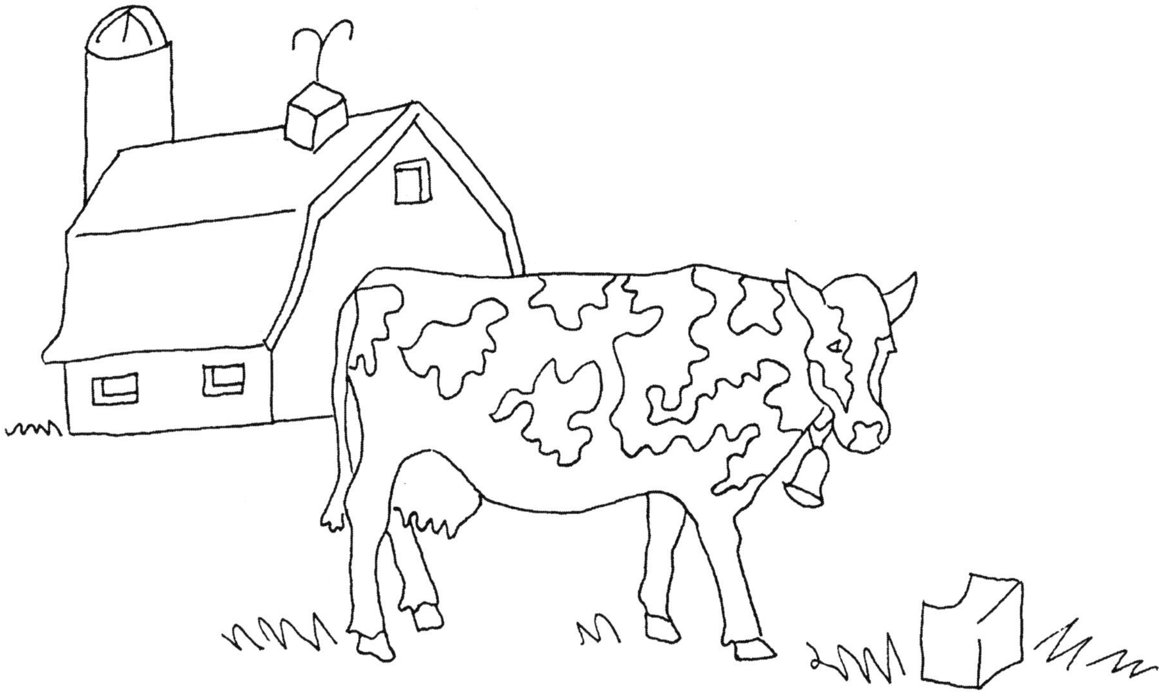

- ❐ The grass is greener on the other side.
- ❐ Don't cry over spilled milk.
- ❐ Children are to be seen and not herd.
- ❐ Take the bull by the horns.
- ❐ Don't be Bossy!
- ❐ Clumsy as a bull in a china closet.
- ❐ Cow-nt your blessings.
- ❐ Don't go to bed in an angry moo-d.

Exercise 74

SWEET MEMORIES

Purpose:

- Share memories and feelings about a common subject to enhance feelings of belonging.
- Promote group support for coping with dietary restrictions and limitations.

Materials:

One photocopy of the illustration for each group member; crayons and pencils.

Procedure:

1. As materials are being passed out, members are asked to think about experiences they have had with ice cream parlors and soda fountains.
2. The leader encourages members to write their favorite ice cream treat in the blank, draw the treat, and color the pictures.

Group Discussion:

Members share memories about the illustration, ice cream parlors, and soda fountains. Each member shows his or her illustration and tells about a favorite ice cream treat. Reminiscing about a nonthreatening subject helps to build group cohesion.

The leader asks if any members have dietary limitations for ice cream, sweets, or other foods. Members who have special dietary needs are asked to tell about their diets and how they feel about the restrictions.

Group support and encouragement is offered to members who express frustrations or resentments about their diets. Sharing feelings about dietary restrictions helps members to handle frustration and learn new ways to cope.

Sweet Memories

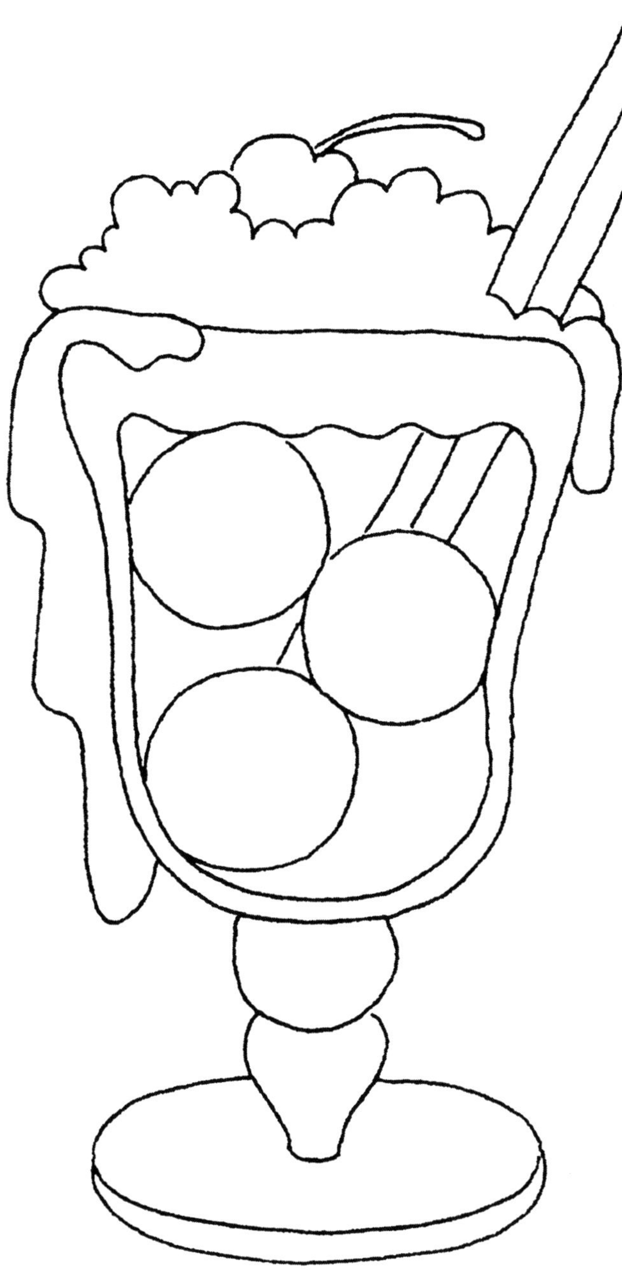

My favorite ice cream treat: ____________________________

____

Exercise 75

FEELING TRAPPED

Purpose:

- Open up feelings of frustration for group support.
- Share ideas on ways to overcome feelings of isolation and entrapment.

Materials:

One photocopy of the illustration for each member; pencils and crayons.

Procedure:

1. Photocopies are distributed and members are asked to identify the picture.
2. The leader or a member describes how a minnow bucket is used to trap minnows which are then used as bait for fishing.
3. Members are asked to think about times in their lives when they have felt trapped and how they handled the situation.
4. Members are asked to complete the sentences below the picture. Members may color the illustration if they wish.

Group Discussion:

Members share their sentences about feeling trapped and describe how they handled the situation. The group leader encourages support by acknowledging that everyone has felt trapped at some time in their lives.

Some members may feel trapped in their present living situation. Ideas for coping and suggestions for feeling less confined are elicited from the group. Sharing frustrations and discussing coping techniques reduces feelings of isolation and helplessness.

Members are asked to share memories about using a minnow bucket or other fishing experiences. Reminiscing about a common subject builds feelings of relatedness and belonging.

Feeling Trapped

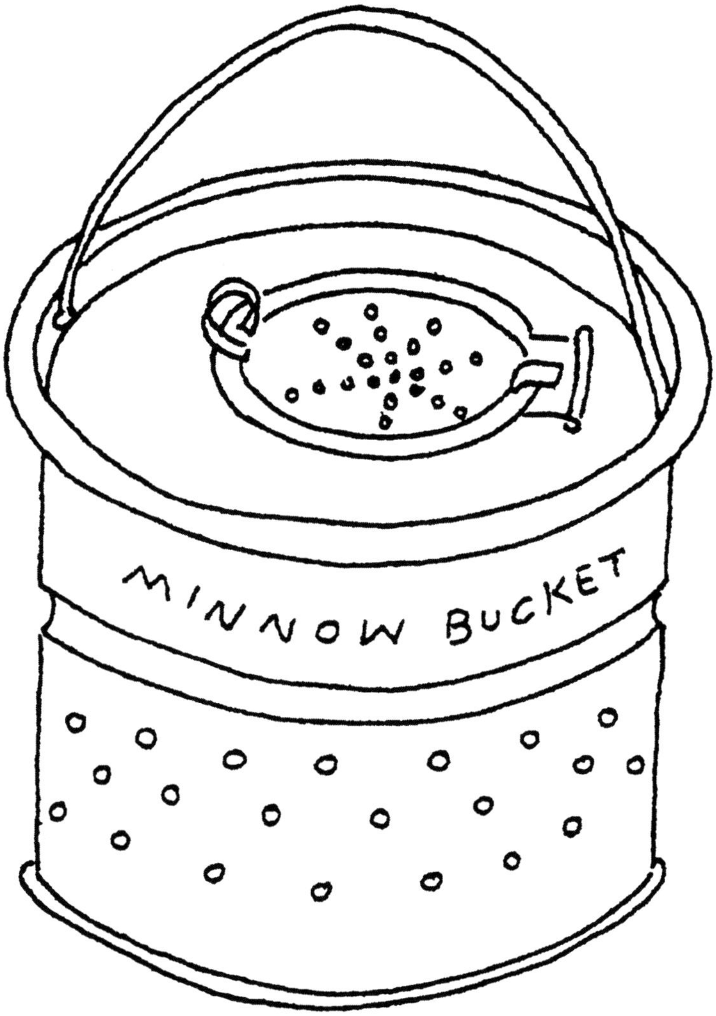

I felt trapped when: ______________________________
____
____

I handled the situation by: __________________________
____
____

Exercise 76

HOLIDAY LETTER

Purpose:

- Improve relatedness by increasing communication.
- Expand awareness of others.

Materials:

One photocopy of the letter for each member; pencils and crayons. ***Optional:*** slips of paper and a hat or box.

Procedure:

1. Materials are distributed and the sentence fragments are read aloud.
2. Members are asked to write, "Dear Group," and fill in the blanks in the rest of the letter. If needed, help is given so that all group members can complete the letter.
3. Members are encouraged to color the picture and add additional holiday designs to the border of the letter if they wish.

Group Discussion:

Members present their illustrations and read their letters to the group. The leader asks group members to share about other special holiday memories.

This exercise is effective in promoting group cohesiveness and encouraging shy members to open up.

Variation:

Members may draw each other's names from a hat and write a letter to the member whose name was drawn. In this variation make sure adequate help and supervision are provided for the letter writing so that each member receives a completed, appropriate holiday letter.

Holiday Letter

Dear ____________________________,

I remember celebrating the holidays by: ______________

____

I especially liked: ___________________________________

____

For a holiday dinner we often had: ___________________

____

Hope your holiday is filled with: ____________________

____

____

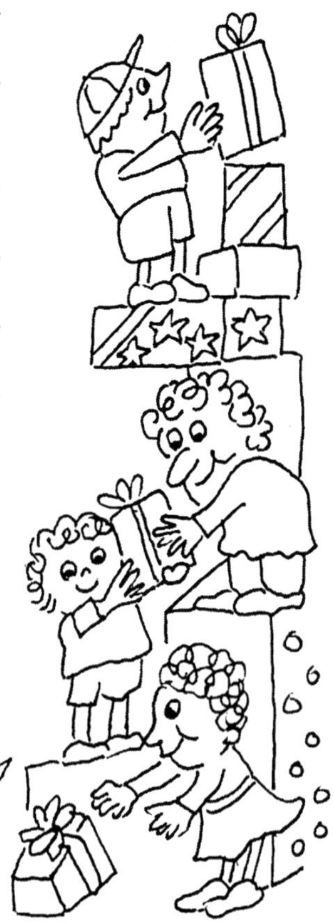

Don't forget to: ________________________

____

____

____

Warm holiday wishes from

____

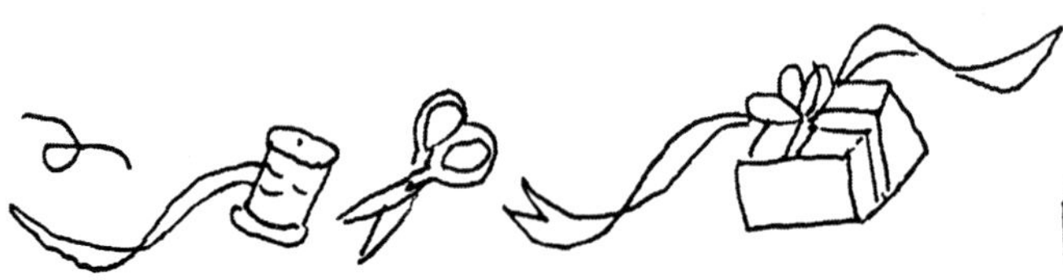

Exercise 77

MEMORIES OF MOTHER

Purpose:

- Increase understanding of self and others by sharing feelings about family.
- Work through unfinished or unresolved feelings about mother or mother figure.

Materials:

One photocopy of the illustration for each member; pencils and fine-line colored felt pens.

Procedure:

1. Members are asked to think about their mother or a mother figure in their lives.
2. Materials are distributed and the sentences are read aloud.
3. Members are asked to complete the sentences.
4. The leader encourages members to draw and color a picture of their mother, or a mother figure in the frame.

Group Discussion:

Members share their pictures and feelings about mother. The leader asks members to share how they are similar or different from their mother. If a group member had no mother figure, that member may share ideas on the mother he or she would like to have had.

This exercise is effective in helping members gain perspective on their relationship with their mother. Members who vent feelings of disappointment about their mothers may be asked to share how they made up for their mothers' deficiencies and what coping skills they used to survive.

Memories of Mother

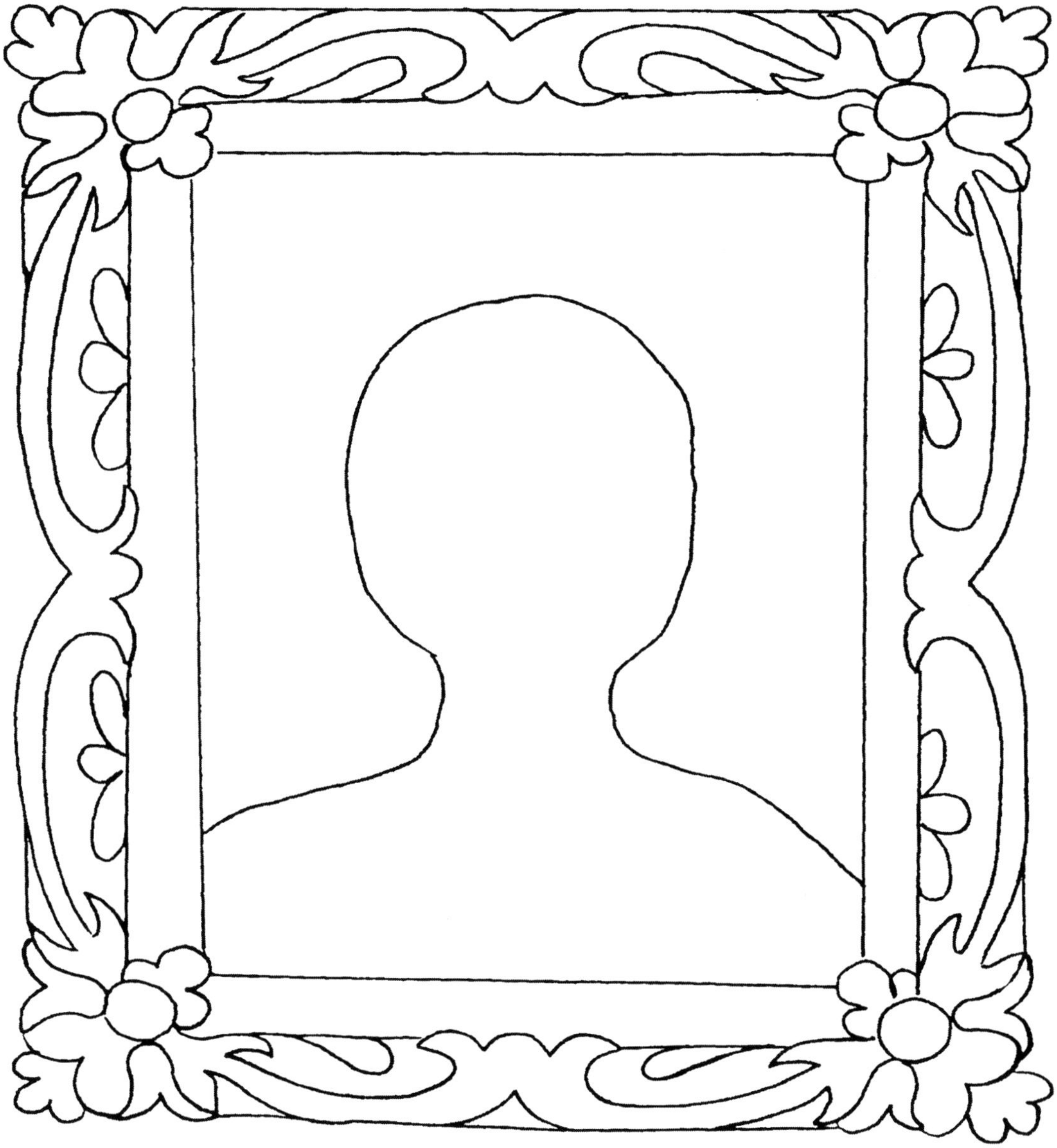

My mother was good at: ______________________________

I liked it when she: ___________________________________

Sometimes I wished she would: _______________________

If I could talk to her today, I'd tell her: ________________

____

Exercise 78

SHARING TRAVELS

Purpose:

- Promote self-disclosure to enhance identity and relatedness.
- Increase awareness of common experiences to increase understanding of others.

Materials:

One copy of the illustration for each member; crayons.

Procedure:

1. Photocopies of the illustration and crayons are passed out to the members.
2. Group leader encourages members to identify points of interest shown on the map and to share about those they have visited or lived near.
3. Members may color in areas of special interest.

Group Discussion:

Members are asked to share about a special vacation or other travel experience they have had or would like to have had.

The leader asks members how they felt about family vacations when they were growing up. Members are asked to describe their role in the family vacation. Members who did not take family vacations are asked to tell what they would like to have done for a vacation. Members are asked to tell whether they planned similar or different vacations later in life.

By sharing about vacations and travel, members may discover common interests and experiences. Sharing personal history of this nature enhances identity and promotes reminiscence.

Sharing Travels

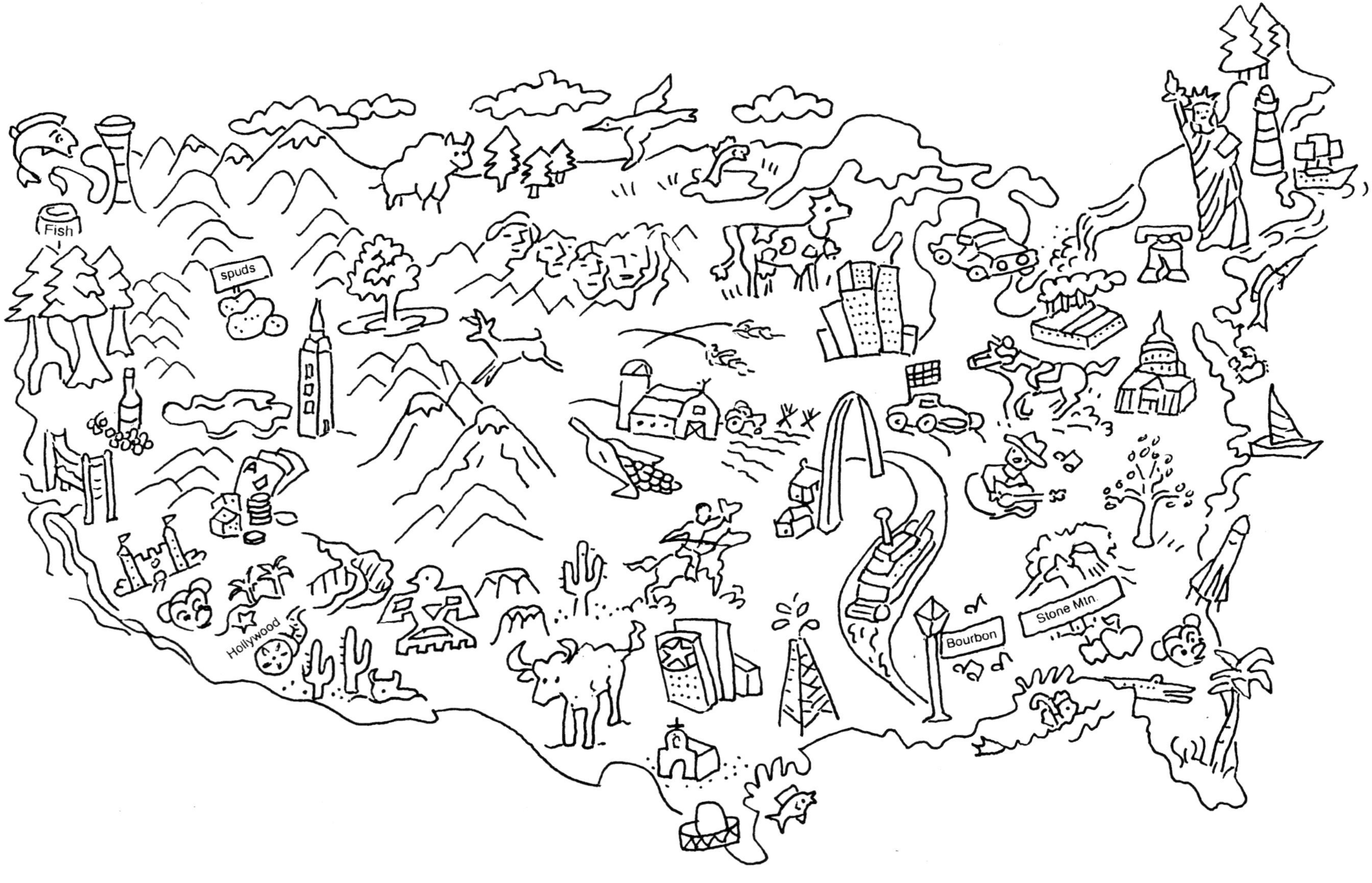

Exercise 79

STEPS TO SELF-ESTEEM

Purpose:

- Raise awareness of ways to increase self-esteem.
- Instill hope by encouraging positive goals.
- Promote group cohesiveness.

Materials:

Photocopy of the illustration for each member; pencils and crayons.

Procedure:

1. Materials are distributed and the leader or a member reads the caption about self-esteem.
2. The leader encourages members to tell about ways to raise self-esteem.
3. Members are instructed to write ideas for improving their own self-esteem on the stair steps.

Group Discussion:

It is important in this exercise that a range of realistic suggestions are made which will encourage members to build self-esteem. Suggestions might include participating in available activities, greeting someone pleasantly at mealtime, or paying special attention to grooming. Each member is asked to choose one idea to try in the next week.

The leader encourages reminiscence by asking members if they have lived in homes with stairways. Members are invited to share memories about stairs, banisters, and under-the-stair closets. Reminiscing about a common subject helps to build trust and group cohesiveness.

Steps to Self-Esteem

Good self-esteem is important in maintaining healthy attitudes and positive ways of coping with life's challenges. When self-esteem is low, it is more difficult to face the problems of daily living. People never outgrow their need to work on strengthening self-esteem.

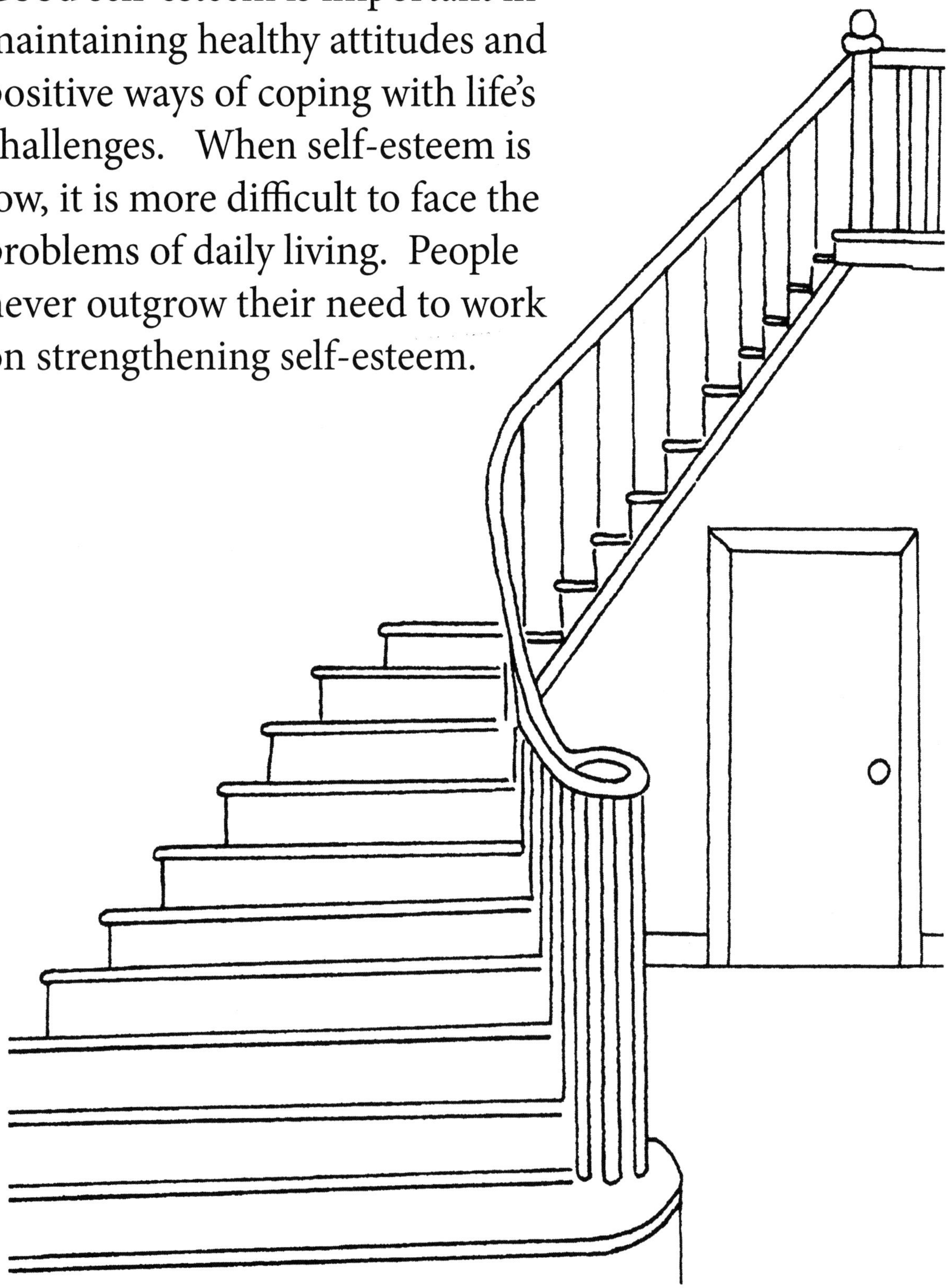

Exercise 80

GIVING THANKS

Purpose:

- Emphasize positive thinking.
- Strengthen identity and self-concept by sharing personal perferences.

Materials:

Old magazines, scissors, glue, felt pens, pencils, and posterboard (orange is effective for a Thanksgiving poster; however, this exercise can be used any time of the year.)

Procedure:

1. Members are asked to cut pictures out of magazines to illustrate something they are thankful for. (If members are unable to use scissors, pre-cut pictures may be provided, or members who can use scissors can be asked to help those members who have difficulty.)
2. Label the poster: "We are thankful for . . . ." Glue the pictures chosen by members on the posterboard. Members are asked to sign their names on the poster beside pictures they have selected. (If a picture cannot be found to represent something a member is thankful for, the idea can be written with felt pen between the pictures.)

Group Discussion:

It is important to broaden the scope of thankfulness as much as possible. Small everyday events and pleasures should not be overlooked, such as coffee in the morning, shelter, a firm mattress, and beautiful sunsets. This exercise may be helpful for members with a negative outlook or those who are suffering from depression. Adding members' names under the pictures they have selected enhances identity and feelings of inclusiveness.

Variations:

Each member is given a photocopy of "We are thankful for . . ." and asked to complete the list. Members may draw pictures in the margins to illustrate their ideas.

We are thankful for. . . .

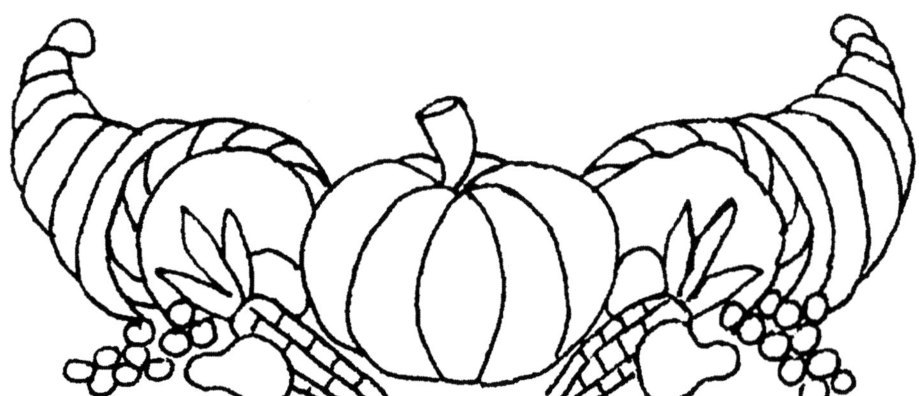

Exercise 81

WELLSPRINGS OF KNOWLEDGE

Purpose:

- Encourage motivation by increasing knowledge of available resources.
- Share background information to promote feelings of belonging.

Materials:

One photocopy of the illustration for each member; pencils and crayons.

Procedure:

1. Materials are distributed and members are asked to share memories and associations to the picture of the well. Some members may recall pumping water, drawing water from a well, or carrying water in long buckets.
2. The sentence fragment on the illustration is read aloud. Members are asked to describe what they think "Wellspring of Knowledge" might refer to. Examples might include knowledgeable people, schools, or libraries.
3. The leader encourages members to think about "Wellsprings of Knowledge" in their own lives and to write their ideas on the blank.
4. Members may color the picture if they wish.

Group Discussion:

Members share their pictures and ideas about "Wellsprings of Knowledge" in their lives.

The leader points out that increasing one's knowledge is a lifetime process. Members are encouraged to tell about subjects they would like to learn more about. The leader and members brainstorm ideas on how to acquire information about the subjects named.

This exercise may enhance motivation and interest in the members' daily life. It is also useful in raising awareness of available resources for learning.

Wellsprings of Knowledge

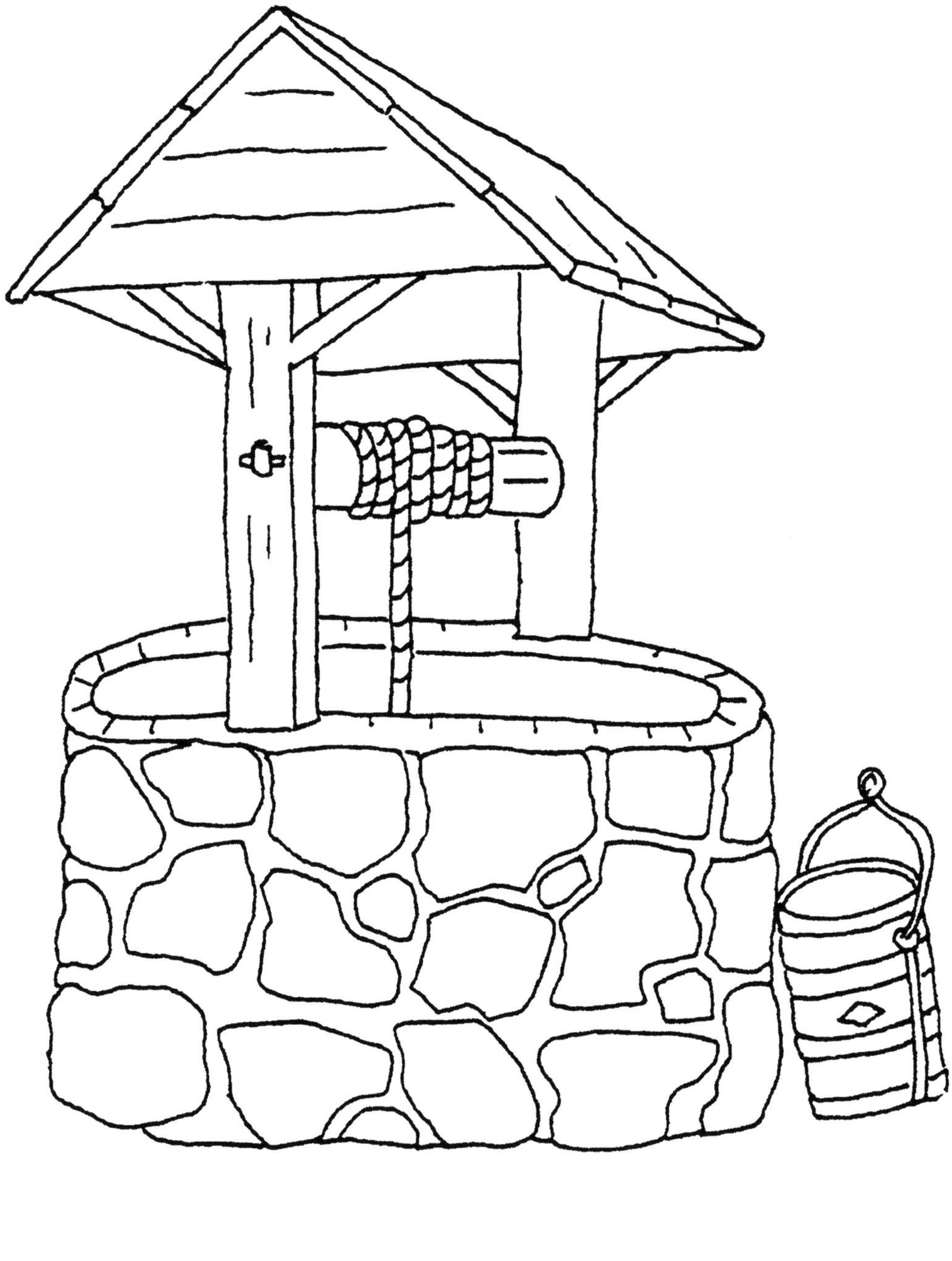

A wellspring of knowledge in my life was: ____________

____

____

Exercise 82

LETTER EXCHANGE

Purpose:

- Promote interaction to increase relatedness.
- Increase awareness of the needs of others.

Materials:

One photocopy of the illustration for each member; pencils and crayons; slips of paper and a hat or box.

Procedure:

1. The leader explains that members are going to write letters to each other. Photocopies of the letter are distributed.
2. Members draw each other's names from a hat.
3. Using the photocopy, each member completes a letter to the member whose name was drawn. Members are asked to volunteer to help those who have difficulty writing so that each member completes a letter.
4. Members may color the illustration if they wish.
5. Members exchange letters.

Group Discussion:

Each member reads their letter and tells how they feel about the letter. The leader asks members to tell how they received mail in the past and whether they ever received a very important letter. Members are encouraged to share memories about the illustrations. Members are asked to describe the current procedure for sending and receiving mail.

This exercise is useful in promoting group cohesiveness. Withdrawn members often feel a greater sense of belonging after they give and receive a group letter.

Letter Exchange

Dear ______________________________,

I'm glad to see you in group because: ________________

____

____

I like your: ____

____

I hope your day is filled with: _______________________

____

____

Thank you for coming to group, and I hope to see you here again.

Warm regards,

____

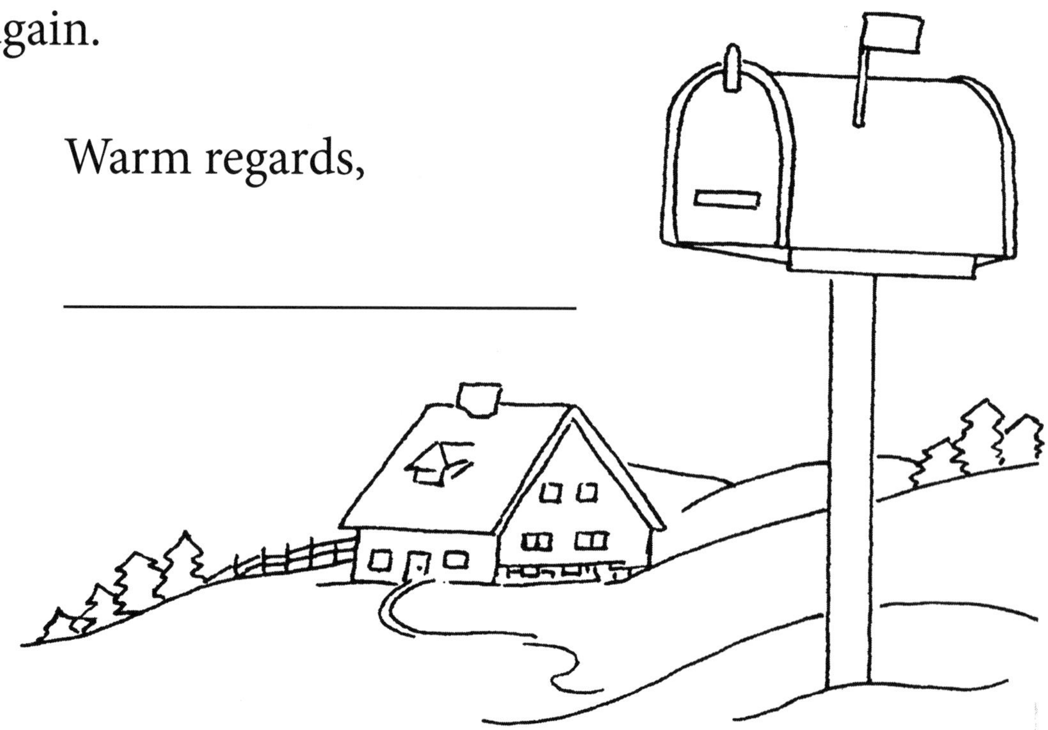

Exercise 83

WEATHERING HARD TIMES

Purpose:

- Reveal personal history to increase feelings of belonging.
- Share stories of survival to emphasize strengths and positive coping.

Materials:

One photocopy of the illustration for each member; fine-line colored felt pens or crayons.

Procedure:

1. While materials are distributed, members are asked to think about storms, floods, hurricanes, or other stressful weather conditions they have experienced.
2. Members are asked to write their worst weather memory in the blank space.
3. Members may color the illustration or draw their own representation of a storm.

Group Discussion:

Members are asked to share memories about difficult weather they have encountered. Those who have colored or drawn show their pictures.

The leader asks each member to name coping skills used to survive fierce weather conditions.

Older adults often rely on coping skills they found useful earlier in life. Exploring these coping skills may help group members feel more effectual in solving current problems.

Weathering Hard Times

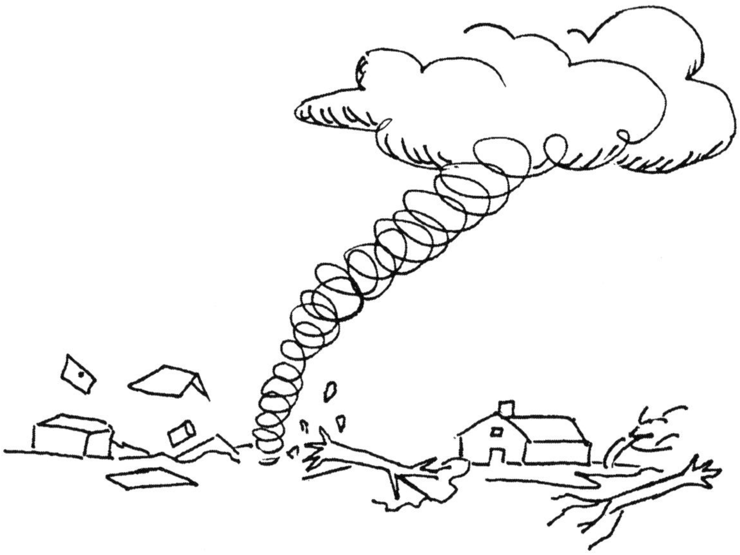

The worst weather condition I have experienced:

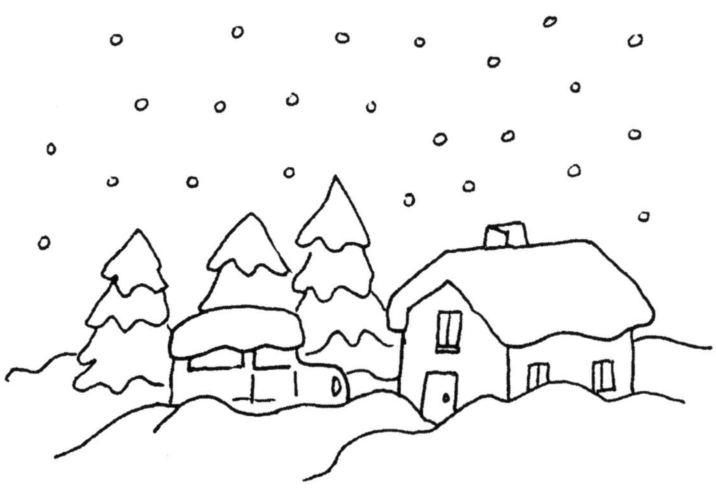

Exercise 84

FRIENDSHIP PIZZA

Purpose:

- Raise awareness of the characteristics of friendly relationships.
- Share personal history of important friendships to increase understanding of others.

Materials:

One photocopy of the illustration for each group member; crayons or colored felt pens, pencils, and scissors. ***Optional:*** posterboard and glue.

Procedure:

1. The leader explains that a good friendship is similar to a good pizza, in that certain ingredients are important.
2. Members are asked to tell what characteristics they think are important to a good friendship.
3. Materials are distributed and the leader tells members that they are going to make a "Friendship Pizza" to illustrate their ideas about friendship.
4. Members are asked to list characteristics of friendship that are important to them on the blanks in their pizza slice. Assistance is given to members who do not write.
5. Members may color the pizza slices if they wish.
6. The pizza slices are cut out and joined into a whole pizza during the discussion described below.

Group Discussion:

Members present their illustrations and ideas about friendship. After each presentation, the member's "pizza slice" is displayed in the center of the table, so that together, the slices form a whole pizza.

Members are asked to share about important friendships they have experienced, including current friendships.

The leader asks members for suggestions on how to encourage friendly attitudes in their present living situation.

Sharing about characteristics of friendship and friendships of the past may raise awareness of current opportunities for relating to others.

Variation:

The pizza slice illustrations can be glued onto posterboard with the title "Friendship Pizza."

Friendship Pizza

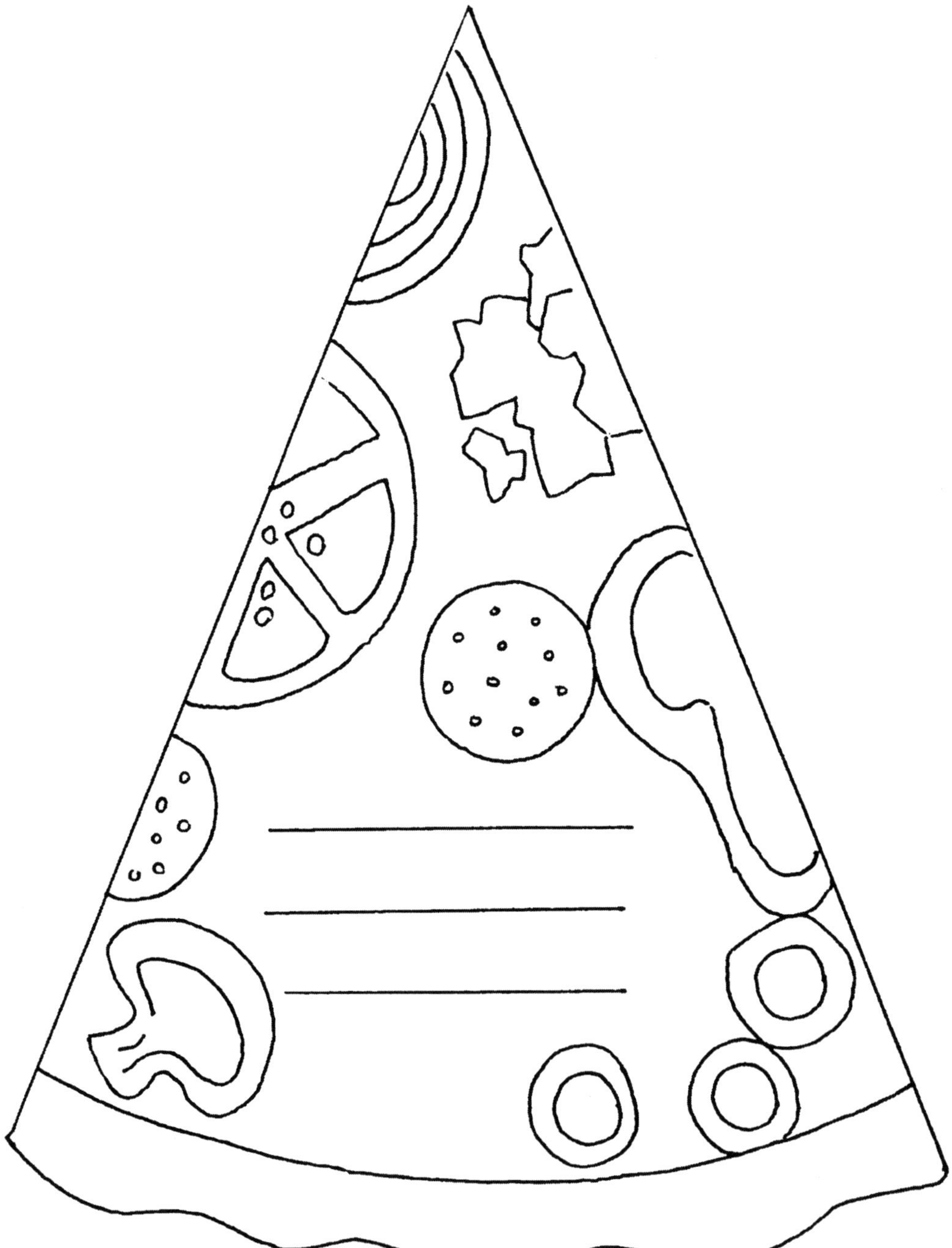

Exercise 85

SCHOOLS DAYS

Purpose:

- Share personal background to increase understanding of self and others.
- Stimulate reminiscence to enhance feelings of identity and self-worth.

Materials:

One photocopy of the illustration for each group member; pencils and crayons.

Procedure:

1. While materials are passed out, members are asked to think about their school experiences.
2. The sentence fragments are read aloud and members are asked to describe the attitudes of the students in the picture.
3. Members are instructed to draw themselves in the empty desk and complete the sentences. Members may color the picture if they wish.

Group Discussion:

Members present their illustrations and sentences. The leader encourages members to share feelings and anecdotes about their school experiences. Members may discover they have feelings or experiences in common which help to build feelings of community. Members are asked if they would approach learning differently if they had it to do over. Current opportunities for learning can be discussed including current events, television, and radio.

School Days

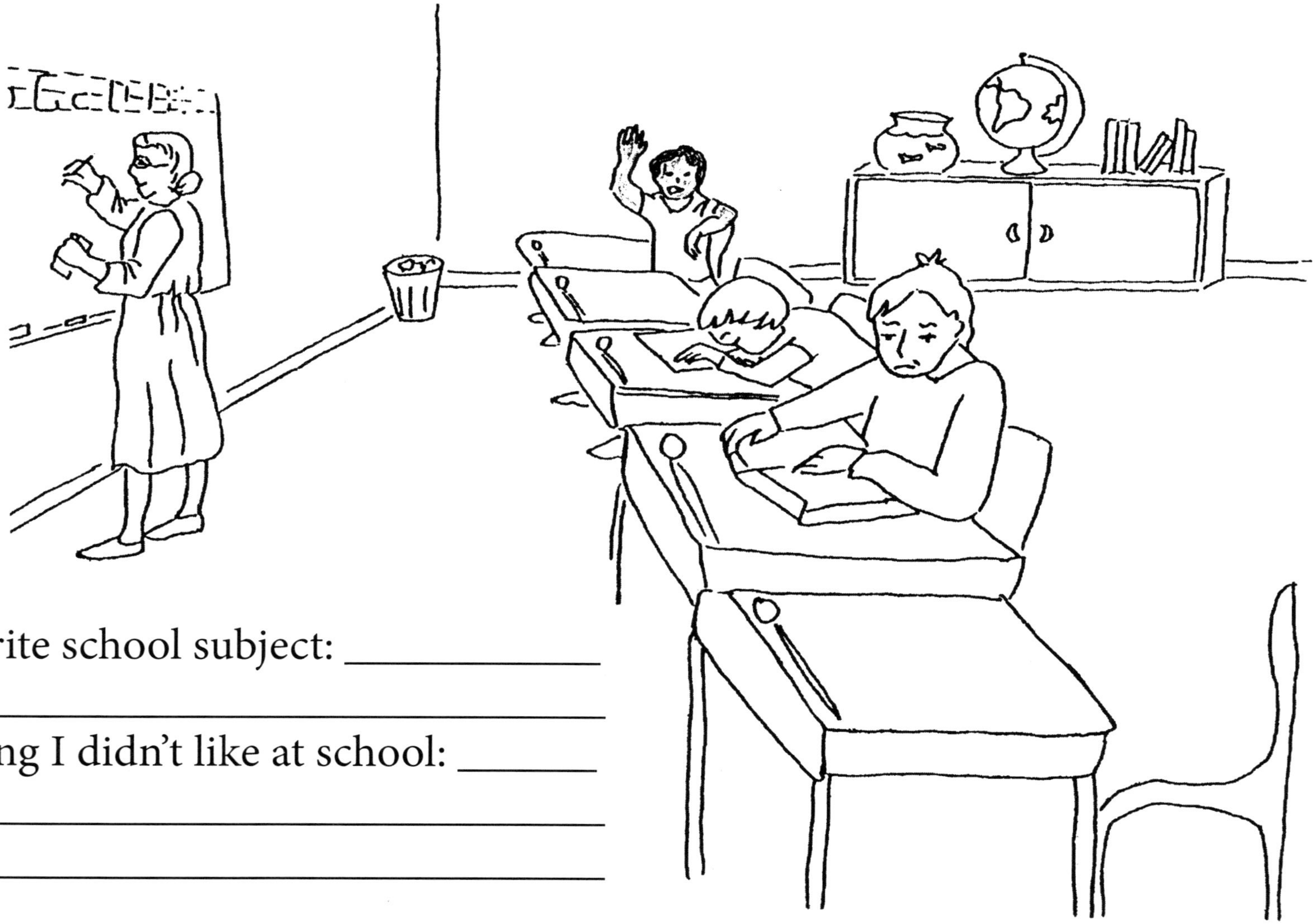

My favorite school subject: ______________

____

Something I didn't like at school: _______

____

____

____